THE
LIVER
CURE

THE

LIVER
CURE

DR. RUSSELL BLAYLOCK, MD
with Charlotte Libov

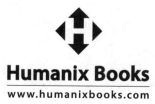

Humanix Books
www.humanixbooks.com

THE LIVER CURE
Copyright © 2022 by Humanix Books

Humanix Books, P.O. Box 20989, West Palm Beach, FL 33416, USA
www.humanixbooks.com | info@humanixbooks.com

Library of Congress Cataloging-in-Publication Data is available upon request.

Humanix Books is a division of Humanix Publishing, LLC. Its trademark, consisting of the words "Humanix Books," is registered in the Patent and Trademark Office and in other countries.

Disclaimer: The information presented in this book is not specific medical advice for any individual and should not substitute medical advice from a health professional. If you have (or think you may have) a medical problem, speak to your doctor or a health professional immediately about your risk and possible treatments. Do not engage in any care or treatment without consulting a medical professional.

ISBN: 9-781-63006-135-7 (Hardcover)
ISBN: 9-781-63006-137-1 (E-book)

Printed in the United States of America
10 9 8 7 6 5 4 3 2 1

This book is dedicated to my youngest grandson, Finn,
who is with the Lord in Heaven. My family's grief
at his loss knows no bounds. Only the Lord comforts us.

I also dedicate this book to my beautiful wife, Diane,
and my two sons: my youngest son, Damien,
a master professional videographer, and my oldest son,
Ron, a master professional photographic artist.

A special dedication to my son Ron and his wife Lindsey,
the parents of our precious Finn Blaylock.

Also, to my other grandchildren, Gabe, Declan, and Susanna.

And finally, to my parents, my wife's parents,
and her dear brother, Ron, who was killed in Vietnam
and is now with the Lord greeting Finn.

Contents

CHAPTER 1

Your Remarkable Liver

M ost medical discussions in the media are concerned with the more glamorous disorders of the body, those that affect the heart, the brain, the lungs, the GI tract, maybe even the kidneys. These rarely include the liver. When the liver *is* mentioned, it usually concerns a viral infection, such as hepatitis B or hepatitis C. As a result, most people know very little about their liver and just how important it really is. Without a liver, we would die very quickly.

One mistake people often make is to assume organs can operate, or do operate, in isolation. We often hear the question— What does the liver do, or the pancreas? We should always keep in mind that all our organs and tissues interact constantly and when one organ fails, many other organs and tissues are adversely affected. And they do communicate with each other. We still do not fully understand the entire extent of this intercommunication, but we know for certain that when one organ, such as the liver malfunctions, other organs will alter their function as well. Ironically, this also includes the brain.

A Quick Look at Your Liver

The liver is the largest organ in the body, weighing in at 1500 grams, or about three pounds, and has a reddish-brown color. For those who remember their geometry, the liver is in the shape of a scalene triangle with the hypotenuse at the bottom. For everyone else, it looks like a wedge, tucked under the ribs on the right side of our bodies. It is partially anchored to the underside of the diaphragm on the right side.

The liver is positioned beneath the rib cage to protect it from injury, which indicates its importance. Normally the lower edge of the liver does not extend below the lowest rib. You may recall that, during a physical examination, your doctor will start pushing on your abdomen just below the ribs on your right side. They do this to get an idea of where the liver's edges are. If your liver is enlarged, its lower edge will be below the lowest rib on the right. The further down the liver protrudes, the greater the doctor's concern, because this could indicate that your liver is enlarged and possibly diseased or malfunctioning.

Your liver is also unusual in that, in addition to the usual blood supply by an artery and a vein, it also has a special blood supply that carries blood from the intestines directly to the liver. This special set of veins is called the **hepatic portal vein system**. Interestingly, this special portal vein supplies 75% of all the blood supplied to the liver. The hepatic portal vein carries nutrients and toxic materials from the intestines, red blood cells and breakdown products of blood cells (old blood cells being removed by the spleen), endocrine secretions from the pancreas, and special endocrine secretions from the gastrointestinal tract to the liver.

Blood within the hepatic portal vein is very poorly oxygenated. The liver can operate with less oxygen than most other organs. Drainage of the liver is rather complex and involves the usual type of veins (hepatic veins) and special sinusoidal capillaries.

This arrangement allows all the cells of the liver to come into direct contact with the blood supply, which is needed for all the intricate functions the liver performs. An additional drainage system is provided by the lymphatics. All these blood vessels make the liver a very vascular organ. Injuries to the liver can result in an extreme danger of bleeding to death.

Interestingly, the liver has one of the highest regeneration abilities of any organ. It can be regenerated if one leaves just one-third undamaged or intact, and it can do so very rapidly. In fact, when the liver re-grows, it grows faster than any cancer, but unlike the cancer, it forms a perfectly functioning new liver replacement, not a tumor.

Your Liver Under the Microscope

If you were to examine your liver under a microscope, you would discover it is composed of numerous lobules, which are tiny six-sided lobes (hexagrams), and within these subdivisions you would find blood vessels, canals (or ducts), and sinusoids, with these vascular spaces being interspersed with liver cells, called **hepatocytes**, which comprise about 55–65% of the organ's mass. While it is these cells that are involved in the liver's main functions, other cells have specialized functions that are also critical. These lobules are designed to allow extensive exposure of the surface of liver cells to the circulating blood, which lets these cells extract nutrients, toxins, and hormones from the circulating blood and secrete all the various products manufactured by the liver cells back into the circulation.

Your liver resembles a massive factory that is constantly working to manufacture and/or store all the proteins, carbohydrates, fats, hormones, several vitamins, iron, and other components your body needs for good health, and especially to protect you from toxic compounds inside your body. The liver never rests. Because the liver plays such an important role in supplying all the nutrients, proteins, and structural components of all the cells in your body, and especially because it is your number-one protection against harmful substances entering your body (and even being produced by your body), it is continually at work. You should make it a point to better understand how the liver affects every other organ in your body—especially your brain. Why? Because your brain is extremely sensitive to toxic substances within the blood circulation, sometimes even when in low concentrations. When the liver fails, we see a progressive loss in function of other organs, such as the heart, the kidneys, the lungs, the pancreas, and the brain.

The Major Roles the Liver Plays

The following is a list of the major functions of the liver, but it is not all-inclusive. We are still discovering other functions it has.

- Nutrient metabolism
  - Proteins
  - Carbohydrates
  - Lipids (Fats)
  - Vitamins/minerals
- Detoxification
  - Pharmaceutical drugs
  - Illicit drugs
  - Food toxins
  - Toxins produced during metabolism or by illness
  - Toxins produced by bacteria in the GI tract
- Nutrient storage
- Immunity

- Blood coagulation
- Cholesterol metabolism
- Bile production
- Endocrine-like functions

Nutrient Metabolism

The liver plays a major role in the metabolism of the food you eat, transforming the carbohydrates, fats, and proteins you consume in your diet into the energy your body needs to function.

It does this by processing the blood that flows to it from the small intestine, breaking down the foods into carbohydrates, fats, and proteins that the body will then use, or store for later. These functions are carried out by the liver cells, called *hepatocytes*, which make up approximately 65% of the cells in the liver.

The liver plays an important role in fat digestion and absorption, as well as absorption of fat-soluble vitamins. It does this by producing bile, which is made up of water, bile salts, cholesterol, and bilirubin. Bilirubin is a substance produced when the liver processes old dead red blood cells. After the bile is produced, it travels through the liver's bile ducts until it reaches the gallbladder, where it is stored to be used when needed. Fats in the upper intestines stimulate the gallbladder to secrete its stored bile into the common bile duct, which empties into the jejunum of the upper small intestine, where it mixes with the partially digested fats. The bile emulsifies the fats, allowing them to be better absorbed.

Bile also aids in absorbing fat-soluble vitamins such as vitamin A, E, and D.

People with gallbladder disease or liver disease will have stool that is white in color and floats in the toilet bowl. This is because of the high levels of undigested fat in the stool. Bile normally imparts the dark brown color to bowel movements. Individuals with liver disorders can also have deficiencies in fat-soluble vitamins.

Occasionally, a person will pass a stool with a bright green sheen to it, which means the gallbladder released a large amount of fresh bile into the intestine before it could become dark. In most cases, it means little in terms of health. This type of discolored stool can be seen with diarrhea or after a fatty meal. If it persists, however, it could mean intestinal problems and you should see your doctor.

The liver also absorbs glucose from your blood and stores it in the liver as glycogen, which is made up of many units of glucose packed together. If your blood sugar falls too low, the liver will break down the glycogen, thus releasing some of the glucose back into the blood stream. We call this process glycogenolysis. Eating a diet very low or devoid of carbohydrates will deplete the liver's glycogen rather rapidly and this increases one's risk of hypoglycemia, especially during vigorous exercise or when under physical stress.

The liver produces most of the body's circulating proteins, known as plasma proteins. These include albumin, lipoproteins such as very low-density lipoproteins (VLDL), high-density lipoproteins (HDL), and low-density lipoproteins (LDL) used for cholesterol transport, and the glycoproteins used in iron transport, such as haptoglobin, transferrin, and hemopexin. Albumin is also important for balancing the water content in blood. Non-immune alpha and beta globulins are produced by the liver and are responsible for the osmotic pressure in the blood and tissues. They are also used to transport various substances in the blood. Liver disorders frequently result in swelling of the extremities, which is caused by a deficiency in albumin. We call this excess tissue fluid edema, which most often appears around the ankles and the face.

The liver also manufactures cholesterol. Because of the health campaigns that targeted cholesterol as a major cause for atherosclerosis, you may have been led to believe that even slightly elevated cholesterol is a bad thing. All scientific studies agree—elevated cholesterol is not the major cause of atherosclerosis, which is what leads to heart attacks and strokes. Your body needs cholesterol for a number of functions, including the production of hormones. In addition, all cell membranes require cholesterol for proper functioning. Low cholesterol levels cause abnormal brain function, especially amnesia and confusion, and major problems can arise from use of cholesterol-lowering drugs.

Under starvation conditions, the liver converts fats into ketones, which better protect the heart and brain. The liver can also convert certain amino acids into fatty acids, for fat storage.

Several vitamins are stored in the liver, including vitamins A, E, K, and B_{12}. Vitamin A is stored as a retinyl ester within special liver cells called **stellate cells**. Vitamin A, which is important for color vision, immune function, transcription of genes, and the transport of iron from the liver, is stored and mobilized from the liver several times a day to keep the blood levels of the vitamin constant.

Vitamin D is also stored in the liver, and in fact, the liver is critical for metabolizing vitamin D into its most active form. Only a relatively small amount of vitamin D is stored in the liver. Thus, taking higher doses of vitamin D will not cause excessive vitamin D buildup. Vitamin E, like vitamin D is stored somewhat in the liver, but not to the extent that we see with vitamin A. Another vitamin stored in the liver is vitamin K, which is critical for blood clotting, acts as a co-enzyme, and reduces inflammation. Very little vitamin B_{12} is stored in the body, with 50% being stored in the liver. With dietary deficiencies, vitamin B_{12} is rapidly depleted.

Several minerals are stored in the liver, such as iron, manganese, magnesium, and copper. Of these, the two most important include iron and copper. Copper is essential for protein and energy production, and low copper levels are associated with oxidative damage to the liver and hepatotoxicity (damage to the liver). Copper, like iron, is a double-edged sword—too little is dangerous, and too much is very dangerous. Another important mineral for the liver is selenium. Deficiencies of this mineral can cause liver necrosis and result in the death of liver cells. Low levels of selenium are common with many chronic diseases. Excessive intake of selenium can also cause toxicity. One should limit their intake to no more than 100 micrograms a day. Zinc is important in protecting the liver from copper toxicity, but like most of these minerals, in higher doses zinc can also be toxic. One should probably limit supplementation to no more than 15 mg a day.

Iron is critical for a great number of metabolic functions, as well as for oxygen transport. Iron is used by the mitochondria for energy production. Other functions include DNA synthesis, stimulation of cell growth, and gene expression. Daily supplementation has been shown to result in high levels of inflammation, lipid peroxidation (oxidation of fats), and excessive iron storage. Taking your iron supplement, if needed, every 3 days instead of every day prevents liver damage by iron. It is also known that having excessive iron storage significantly worsens liver damage by nonalcoholic fatty liver disease and can result in insulin resistance, which plays a major role in many chronic diseases. Iron is stored in the hepatocytes as ferritin.

In the genetic disorder hemochromatosis, one sees excess iron storage in the liver, which over time can result in liver cirrhosis and eventual liver failure. It also increases the risk of developing liver cancer. In this condition, vitamin C supplementation can further increase iron absorption, greatly worsening the condition.

The liver also plays a role in metabolizing several of the hormones. For example, the thyroid gland secretes thyroid hormone in the form of T4 which is converted in the liver to the more active form T3. A similar process occurs with growth hormone. Growth hormone plays a major role in regeneration of the liver during liver injuries. Growth hormone, along with insulin-like growth factor-1 (IGF-1), also reduces liver fibrosis (scarring), reduces dramatically visceral fat accumulation (most often associated with cardiovascular diseases, insulin resistance, and poor health), and protects the liver from fat accumulation, as seen with nonalcoholic fatty liver disease and nonalcoholic steatohepatitis (NAFLD and NASH), respectively. Both insulin and glucagon are degraded in the liver.

Detoxification

While detoxification takes place in all cells in the body, the three major sites of detoxification are the kidneys, the gastrointestinal tract, and the liver. I will limit my discussion to liver detoxification. Most detoxification within the liver takes place within the hepatocyte cells, which make up the bulk of the cells in the liver. You will recall they are arranged in radiating columns within the six-sided lobules, so they are maximally exposed to the blood circulating through the liver, which allows these cells to remove the toxic substances from the blood for processing and ultimate removal from the body.

Liver detoxification takes place by two metabolic systems called **phase I** and **phase II** detoxification. Phase I is the first line of defense against xenobiotics (substances not natural to the body, such as toxic substances and drugs), steroids, various hormones, and pharmaceutical drugs. To carry out this detoxification, in **phase I detoxification** these cells utilize a number of enzymes called **CYP-450 enzymes**. These enzymes all have names that begin with **CYP**. Each performs a special detoxification job, even though there is a lot of overlap in how they function.

Linked closely to the phase I system is the phase II system, which is the most important part of detoxification. Phase I creates compounds that are water insoluble, and as a result, they linger in the liver. If they are not removed, many can damage the liver cells. The main job of phase I detoxification is to convert these water-insoluble compounds into water-soluble compounds. In doing this, these potentially toxic compounds can be quickly removed from the body by the kidneys via the urine and through the gastrointestinal tract by way of the bile released from the liver into the intestines.

Most often we think of liver detoxification as dealing with pharmaceutical drugs or poisons from the environment. These are very important, and in these modern times detoxification of environmental chemicals is more important than ever. In 1989 alone, 1000 newly synthesized compounds were introduced into the market—that is, three new chemicals a day. In this same year, over five million pounds of chemical pollutants were introduced into the environment. Not surprisingly, 3 million severe pesticide poisonings and 220,000 deaths have been reported worldwide each year.

While these figures certainly appear shocking, things have only gotten worse. It is estimated that, in 2020, some 385 million cases of poisonings by pesticides occurred among farmers alone, with 11,000 farmers dying due to the exposure. This equates to 44% of all farmers in the world. In the year 2012, approximately 193,000 people died from unintentional poisoning. A great deal of this toxic exposure comes from Roundup, the weed killer. The main ingredient in Roundup is glyphosate, which is now being detected in most foods, water supplies, soft drinks, and even vaccines. Roundup itself is considered to be 125 times more toxic than glyphosate and is the most toxic agricultural and domestically used chemical agent.

While environmental poisoning is of great concern, most people are not aware that their own body makes massive amounts of internal poisons as well. Every day some 50 billon cells in our body die—that's one million cells a second. This means that a little over 3 pounds of your cells are dying each day, which is necessary to make room for new, healthier cells. Yet, you may wonder, where do these dead cells go? Your immune cells, especially neutrophils and macrophages, gobble up most, so that their components can be used to make new cells—sort of like garbage recycling. Yet, a considerable amount of harmful toxic components is also released into the blood stream and lymphatics and is carried to the liver, where they are detoxified. Cell debris is filtered out by the liver and removed by the phagocytic immune cells stationed within the liver.

People suffering chronic diseases or major injuries can release very high levels of damaged cells and their toxic components, which can worsen their condition. In fact, during chemotherapy and/or radiation treatment of cancerous tumors, we may see so many of these toxic cell components released that they result in the death of the person.

I will discuss detoxification in more detail in Chapter 2.

More on Pharmaceutical Drug Metabolism

Nearly half of all Americans have taken at least one prescription drug over the past 30 days, and that doesn't take into consideration the vast amounts of over-the-counter drugs people use.

The fact that these drugs work in our bodies at all can be attributed to the actions of your liver. It is your liver that processes these drugs, but although it is the processing by our liver that makes these drugs work, these altered chemicals can also have toxic effects. This is indeed a delicate balancing act.

Most of the drugs you ingest, whether prescription or over-the-counter, must be metabolized, or broken down, in order to work. Your liver contains the enzymes to do this, by converting them into a form your body can use more effectively or rendering them less toxic so they can be safely excreted.

Of all the metabolic enzymes, the ones produced by the cytochrome P450 (CYP450) gene group (Phase I) are the most important, because they make up 70 to 80% of the enzymes involved in drug metabolism. Some people can have a genetic variant (called a *single nucleotide polymorphism* or *SNP*) or mutation that affects their body's ability to metabolize certain drugs. People with these genetic mutations in their detoxification enzymes are at a greater risk when taking pharmaceutical drugs that require a particular enzyme for detoxification. They are often referred to as "slow metabolizers."

Some drugs are made much more toxic by the liver's detoxification system itself. In other words, the liver makes the drug much more toxic than it would have been otherwise. A good example is acetaminophen (Tylenol), which is made much more toxic by the liver's Phase I detoxification system. Acetaminophen is one of the more toxic drugs in use and accounts for a significant number of people needing a liver transplant. This drug is the leading cause for calls to the Poison Control Center (with over 100,000 calls a year) and is responsible for 56,000 emergency room visits a year.

Incredibly, over 50% of all instances of acute liver failure in this country are secondary to acetaminophen liver damage. Most of these unfortunate individuals will require a liver transplant. Even low doses of this drug can result in liver failure in certain individuals. It also damages the liver and kidneys by dramatically lowering glutathione levels, which make cells highly vulnerable to severe damage by free radicals. In my opinion, this drug should be taken off the market.

Drug metabolism is also affected by any underlying conditions you may have, such as chronic liver or kidney disorders or advanced heart failure.

These factors affect how quickly drugs are metabolized, thus affecting the rate your body clears drugs. Impaired metabolism means that the drug will linger in your body, which when you take your next dose of the medication could cause harm by raising the dose to dangerous levels, since the first dose was not completely cleared. Even a single impaired detoxification enzyme can make certain drugs very dangerous to take. Because certain foods and plant extracts can suppress these detoxification enzymes, one must be careful when combining pharmaceutical drugs with certain foods and natural products.

As you will learn in Chapter 2, certain foods and plant extracts can modulate these detoxification enzymes, meaning they adjust the enzymes to be more effective as needed, rather than just suppressing the enzymes or stimulating them.

Storage

Another job of your liver is to store vitamins A, D, E, and K, as we saw with glycogen and fatty acids, which can then be used by your body as needed. Your liver does this to protect your body in times of nutrient shortage and starvation, so your body can live off these stored nutrients for a relatively long time. In addition, your liver also stores vitamins and minerals that are needed for metabolism, and also to repair cells and tissues.

Immunity

The liver is an important part of the immune system. The inside of the body has two main sites of contact with the outside world—the linings of the lungs and the GI tract. Things we eat, as well as putting contaminated objects in our mouths, allow bacteria, viruses, and fungi to enter the lower gastrointestinal tract. The highest concentration of immune cells is within the walls of the GI tract and passages in the respiratory system (nasopharynx, trachea, and lungs). If these microorganisms get past this first line of defense in the intestines, they are then carried by the hepatic portal circulatory system directly to the liver. The liver contains one of the highest concentrations of phagocytic immune cells in the body, which gobble up these microorganisms like a hungry shark. If conditions worsen, the liver can mount a typical immune attack, just like other areas of the body.

New research is also linking the immune system with longevity. It's known that, as we age, the immune system becomes weaker in terms of its ability to kill invading microorganisms. Ironically, at the same time, the malfunctioning immune system can greatly increase inflammation within the older person's body. High levels of inflammation can occur in the face of poor immune function. This state of affairs with aging is why vaccines do not work in the elderly and can actually make things much worse by worsening the inflammation, while not actually stimulating functional immunity.

As you'll see, good nutrition is important to all immune function. This includes not only adequate protein, carbohydrate, and fat intake, but also all of the vitamins and minerals, especially:

- Vitamin C
- Natural vitamin E (mixed tocopherols and tocotrienols)
- B-complex vitamins
- Carotenoids
- Magnesium
- Zinc

- Selenium
- Manganese
- Magnesium
- Copper

Of specific importance is the finding that even a single deficiency, such as thiamine (B_1), riboflavin (B_2), or pyridoxine (B_6) can cause significant impairment of immune function.

There is also evidence that even low-to-normal levels (subclinical deficiencies) of these critical nutrients can impair immunity.

The medical profession rarely addresses these important, life-saving findings. What this means is that nutritional supplementation can make the difference between a healthy life or poor health, and, in many cases, death.

During infections, the body must produce trillions of white blood cells (lymphocytes, neutrophils, macrophages, and monocytes) to fight the invading microorganisms.

Producing so many cells requires higher levels of vitamins and minerals, as well as adequate amounts of proteins. But it is difficult to replace lost nutrients when an infection is rampant. Rather, it is better to keep your body healthy and well supplied with nutrients in anticipation of a possible infection. And this includes keeping your nutrient stores adequate within the liver.

Protecting Your Brain and Keeping It Sharp

One of your liver's most important jobs is to keep toxins, or poisons, from building up in your blood. When your liver isn't working as well as it should, in severe liver disease, for example, these toxins can build up in your bloodstream and alter the function of your brain. This can cause changes in the way you act, sleep, and also your mood. Such problems can occur suddenly, or gradually, over time.

Mild changes can occur as depression, anxiety, or difficulty focusing, but as the disease progresses—and the toxins build up—symptoms such as hand tremors, jerking muscles or spasms, loss of balance, confusion or disorientation, and difficulty concentrating can occur.

Such confusion and disorientation are commonly referred to as brain fog. Brain fog can occur in people whose livers are not impaired, such as people who are frail or have chronic inflammatory conditions, so it seems obvious that keeping the liver in good shape could help those with other ailments stay sharp.

CHAPTER 2

Detoxification

How the Liver Keeps You Safe and Healthy

We hear a lot about "detox," which is lingo for detoxification. Detoxification can mean a lot of things to different people. Eating a healthy diet is a loose definition of detoxification. In fact, this is not only a first line of defense against food-based toxic substances; it can also stimulate detoxification mechanisms within the various tissues and cells to clean the body of these harmful compounds.

All cells contain some form of detoxification mechanisms, such as special molecules like **glutathione**, which not only act as a powerful antioxidant molecule but can bind and remove several toxic metals, such as lead, mercury, and cadmium. **Metallothionein** is another cellular detoxification molecule that removes harmful metals, including mercury, cadmium, lead, and arsenic.

Other major detoxification systems, as mentioned in Chapter 1, include the kidneys and the cells lining the gastrointestinal tract (GI tract). The cells lining the GI tract are especially important as they form a frontline defense against toxic compounds that can enter the body with eating and drinking.

The liver remains the main detoxification center for the body. It cleans the circulation of toxic substances that not only enter the body from the GI tract, but that are inhaled into the lungs or absorbed from the skin. In fact, absorption of toxic compounds from the skin is a major way these harmful compounds enter the body. It was only fairly recently that it was appreciated just how many harmful substances are absorbed through the skin. This can occur from the use of various skin creams, contamination from pesticide and herbicide sprays, and medications applied to the skin. These substances are rapidly absorbed through the skin and widely distributed in the body. The liver filters these toxic substances out of the blood and renders them less toxic or speeds their elimination from the body. But because these toxic substances are not coming from the GI tract with its direct line to the liver, the liver is less efficient in neutralizing these harmful substances as they circulate through the body before getting to the liver.

Now let's dive deeper into how the liver detoxifies these harmful compounds. As you learned in Chapter 1, the liver uses a two-tier system to deal with these harmful compounds—called *phase I* and *phase II detoxification*.

Phase I Detoxification

We learned in Chapter 1 that the liver uses a large number of detoxification enzymes classified under the grouping CYP-450 enzymes (sometimes just called *P-450 enzymes*). Chemicals are poisonous because of certain ways their molecules are structured, which can be very exacting. To make them less toxic, the liver will chemically alter these toxic compounds so they can do no harm.

The phase I enzymes are the first line of defense—but it is not perfect. Keep in mind, when the liver was created, no artificial chemicals made by pharmaceutical and chemical companies were circulating in the environment. These are new to the liver, which explains why sometimes the phase I enzymes, instead of making these new chemicals less toxic, can make them even more toxic or even carcinogenic (cancer causing).

Normally, the liver's CYP-450 enzymes will attempt detoxification by adding certain chemical groups to the toxic compound to make it less toxic. These include attaching hydroxyl, carboxyl, and amino chemical groups to the toxic molecule. This involves a lot of basic chemistry, so I will spare you all that. Suffice it to say that for 90% of the drugs we are exposed to, this system works very efficiently.

Pharmaceutical drug makers knew that the drugs they were making would be processed by the liver's chemical factory, so they made allowances for whatever changes the liver would make to their drugs. Most importantly, they calculated how long it would take the liver enzymes to neutralize and dispose of the drug in question. For example, if they gave a drug such as Dilantin, the antiseizure drug, they had to know just how long the liver would let it stay in the body until the liver disposed of it. In that way, the pharmaceutical company scientists could determine how often the drug would need to be given to keep blood levels functionally elevated—that is, effective.

For example, if it took 6 hours for the drug to be metabolized and removed by the liver, the doctor would have to prescribe that the drug be given every 6 hours to make it effective. Studies have shown that specific classes of these CYP enzymes are responsible for removing or detoxifying particular drugs. Importantly, it is also known that certain foods, plant extracts, and herbs can alter the efficiency of these detoxifying enzymes.

Let us say that an herb designated as R suppressed the detox-ification enzyme CYP1, which is responsible for removing a par-ticular antibiotic. Normally, the antibiotic would be given every 6 hours, based on how long it took the normal liver to metabolize the antibiotic. But if the person was taking herb R that suppressed the detoxification enzyme CYP1, then the antibiotic would be around longer than the usual 6 hours. So, when the next dose of the antibiotic was taken on schedule, at 6 hours, a lot more of the antibiotic would remain from the first dose. Taking the next dose at that time would mean that you would now be getting far too much of the drug—which could be toxic.

The opposite can also happen when a natural supplement stimulates a detoxification enzyme. This time, let us suppose the medication is an antiseizure drug. Now herb Z stimulates the enzyme that gets rid of the antiseizure drug so it works a lot faster. Normally, the antiseizure medication is given every 8 hours, because that is how long it takes the detoxification enzyme to get rid of the medication. If the person takes their medication as prescribed—that is, every 8 hours—all will be well, because the blood levels of the antiseizure medication will be high enough at all times to stop any seizure from happening, until the next dose of the medication.

But if they take herb Z at the same time, the seizure medica-tion level in the blood will run out before the 8 hours is up—let's say it is now mostly gone by 4 hours. That means at 4 hours after the first dose they will not have a sufficient amount of the anti-seizure medication in their blood to prevent the seizure from hap-pening. As a result, the patient has a major seizure. Not knowing the effect of herb Z, the patient will be puzzled, since they were taking their medication as prescribed.

Most pharmacists have a list of such drug-supplement inter-actions, so that such things will not happen.

In nature, we see many procarcinogenic compounds—that is, chemicals that do not cause cancer as is, but must be chemically converted to cause cancer. They are often converted to cancer-causing compounds by the liver's phase I detoxification system. We see this with a number of pesticides, herbicides, and fungicides, and even with natural carcinogens such as aflatoxin. Your liver is converting these procarcinogens into powerful cancer-causing compounds. For example, the detoxification enzyme CYP1 can convert polycyclic aromatic hydrocarbons (PAH), heterocyclic aromatic amines, and polychlorinated biphenyls (PCBs) into fully carcinogenic compounds.

To get an idea just how important the effectiveness of these enzymes can be, when we see low levels of the detoxification enzyme CYP1A2 in a young male, we know that men with this defect have a much higher incidence of developing testicular cancer.

We also see a strong connection between certain detoxification enzyme defects and neurodegenerative diseases. For example, a defect in CYP2D is associated both with a higher incidence of lung cancer and Parkinson's disease. As you'll recall from Chapter 1, I mentioned certain genetic defects called **single nucleotide polymorphisms** (SNP), which can cause a single enzyme not to function properly. Some of the more common genetic defects involving detoxification enzymes include CYP2C and CYP2D. People with these gene defects are called "poor metabolizers" and have great difficulty detoxifying various pharmaceutical drugs, especially drugs that regulate the heart's rhythm, antiseizure drugs, and warfarin, which is a blood thinner. People with this problem must be careful taking these medications—they must follow altered drug schedules. That is, they have to take the medications further apart than normally prescribed.

Another phase I enzyme, CYP2E1, metabolizes anesthetics such as halothane and isoflurane. Such a defect could cause these individuals to encounter difficulty when undergoing a general anesthetic.

While phase I detoxification works well most of the time, as we have seen, sometimes it makes errors and actually makes things worse—even deadly. The situation with acetaminophen (Tylenol) is a case in point—phase I detoxification can cause this drug to do considerable damage to the liver and kidneys and can even totally destroy the liver.

In cases where phase I enzymes make things worse, we may want to inhibit the enzyme responsible. For example, several flavonoids can significantly interfere with the detoxification enzymes that make acetaminophen toxic, namely, CYP2E1. One of the more effective naturally occurring compounds is kaempferol, which powerfully prevents damage to the liver via several mechanisms. Curcumin is also a powerful liver protector against many toxic substances.

As discussed in the previous chapter, the liver has a powerful backup system for problems such as this. This backup system is the phase II system, which operates in tandem with phase I, but using a different series of mechanisms.

Phase II Detoxification

We learned that phase I detoxification reduced most of the toxicity of dangerous compounds circulating in our blood by a process of oxidation—that is, adding compounds that reduce the toxicity. Unfortunately, this also made the toxic chemicals water insoluble, which could be a big problem because they linger in the liver where they could cause considerable damage.

To prevent this, phase II detoxification changes these toxic substances chemically to make them water soluble. By doing this, these toxic compounds can be eliminated from the body by the kidneys via the urine and through the gastrointestinal tract via the bile.

In chemical language, we call phase II detoxification: conjugation. What this means is a chemical process where special chemicals are added to the toxic compound to make it water soluble. These water-soluble chemicals use special enzymes to perform this process. These include:

- Glucuronic acid (glucuronyl transferases)
- Sulfate (sulfotransferases)
- Glutathione (glutathione transferases)
- Amino acids (amino acid transferases)
- Acetyl groups (N-acetyl transferases)
- Methyl groups (N- and O-methyltransferases)

When our liver faces a particularly heavy toxic load—for instance, when we have eaten a lot of junk food or foods contaminated with high concentrations of agrichemicals—our liver increases the concentration of these phase II detoxification enzymes to handle the new load. The same is true with internal toxic compounds, such as when we are sick, exercise strenuously, or are injured. In all such cases, the blood becomes contaminated with significantly more dead cells than usual, along with harmful metabolic products.

Keep in mind that our hormones are also constantly subjected to metabolism by the liver, and when the liver is functioning abnormally, our hormones are also affected. Under specific circumstances, this can raise our risk of certain hormone-dependent cancers, such as prostate and breast cancers. These detoxification enzymes also change during pregnancy, old age, and living in an environment with high levels of pollution. Many toxic substances can even damage some of the detoxification enzymes, thus impairing efficient detoxification of other dangerous compounds.

Recently, researchers discovered that having an impairment of specific types of glucuronyl transferase enzymes can greatly increase a person's risk of colon cancer. This discovery demonstrates just how important these detoxification enzymes really are. Studies are also showing that having impairment of specific types of these detoxification enzymes can greatly increase a person's risk of developing certain neurodegenerative diseases, such as Parkinson's disease.

A number of studies have shown that exposure to pesticides, herbicides, and certain fungicides can greatly increase a person's risk of developing Parkinson's disease, especially if they have a defect in one of these enzymes. This effect was dramatically demonstrated in a report in a medical journal that described an unfortunate woman who decided to clear her house of insects by spraying everything in sight with a household insecticide. Soon afterward, she developed a very rapid onset of advanced Parkinson's disease.

She was admitted to a local hospital and the neurologist confirmed that she was indeed suffering from advanced Parkinson's, which was unusual because advanced cases can take decades to develop. Over a short period, she recovered completely and returned home. Her family thoroughly cleaned her house before she returned. Immediately on reentering her home, all her Parkinson's symptoms returned. She was hospitalized again, and once again she recovered. Convinced the house was beyond any hope of removing the insecticide, she and her husband moved to a new home free of contamination. She did well until her family brought her one of her blouses from the old house. Once she put it on, all her symptoms returned.

Most notably, this never happened to her husband, even though he lived in the same house, and none of her relatives experienced any problems when visiting the house. It was concluded that the poor lady had a defect in one or more detoxification enzymes needed to detoxify the insecticide, and, as a result, even extremely small amounts of the bug spray caused her to develop advanced Parkinson's disease–like symptoms.

One of the strongest links to Parkinson's disease is chronic exposure to pesticides, herbicides, and fungicides. The reason appears to be that they can overwhelm the liver's ability to detoxify these harmful chemicals. People born with certain genetic defects (single nucleotide polymorphisms or SNPs) affecting specific detoxification enzymes are much more susceptible to such chemically induced neurodegenerative diseases. As we age, the liver's ability to detoxify these poisons can become impaired as well. This puts us at a high risk of harm by being exposed, not only to environmental poisons, but also to the toxic substances produced by our own body.

Sulfotransferase enzymes are another method used in the phase II system to make toxic compounds water soluble. Here sulfur groups are chemically bonded to these toxic substances. This type of detoxification is important for metabolizing hormones, such as thyroid hormone, estrogens, and androgens. The sulfur-containing amino acids, especially taurine, are particularly important for supporting this type of detoxification. Garlic and onions are also an important source of these sulfur compounds.

Another part of phase II detoxification utilizes a chemical called *glutathione-S-transferase*. Regularly taking acetaminophen can drastically lower glutathione levels, which will deplete this important detoxification system. The transfer of acetyl chemical groups to toxic compounds is important for detoxifying certain drugs containing hydrazines or aromatic amines, such as isoniazid, hydralazine, and sulfonamides. Defects in this detoxification enzyme can result in a high incidence of drug reactions, resulting in liver damage.

Finally, several natural compounds contribute a methyl group for detoxification of potentially toxic compounds and for metabolizing estrogens. The amino acid methionine, vitamins B_{12}, B_6, folate, and betaine are important for supporting this form of detoxification. You may recall the craze with taking a product called *SAMe* for depression. SAMe (S-adenosyl-L-methionine) is also a methyl donor used in detoxification.

Foods, Plant Extracts, and Other Nutritional Supplements Affecting Detoxification

Several vegetables and plant extracts can alter the various enzymes used for detoxification by the liver. When dealing with certain plant extracts or components, it is important to appreciate that the dose is essential, as for some compounds, such as curcumin, an extract from the spice turmeric, a low dose stimulates the phase I enzyme CYP1A1, whereas a higher dose suppresses it—which may be good or bad, depending on the situation. To prevent a procarcinogen from being converted into a fully active carcinogen, one may want to suppress certain detoxification enzymes. Under such circumstances, a higher dose of curcumin would be advantageous. Celery also inhibits this enzyme.

Under most circumstances, this is a good thing because it prevents your phase I enzymes from producing cancer-causing compounds. Yet, suppressing a detoxification enzyme would be harmful if a particular pharmaceutical drug requires this enzyme for its metabolism. Even then, it is all a matter of reducing the dose of the medication or changing scheduling as far as how often to take the drug.

Sometimes it's all a matter of the total effect of a food or plant extract. For example, cruciferous vegetables (kale, Brussels sprouts, and broccoli) and resveratrol (and resveratrol-containing plants) can induce this same enzyme, but these plants contain a number of anticancer compounds that easily override any effect of stimulating this detoxification enzyme.

In many of these studies of the effects of plants or plant extracts, the researchers used very high doses, far beyond what a person would normally consume. Yet, we should not ignore these interactions, especially when dealing with pharmaceutical drugs.

Other commonly consumed food items that can affect phase I detoxification include rooibos tea, garlic, fish oil, green tea, black tea, and quercetin. These supplement compounds all affect one of the more clinically important detoxification enzymes called *CYP3A enzymes*. These groups of enzymes are used to detoxify caffeine, testosterone, progesterone, and the carcinogen aflatoxin B_1. It also is responsible for detoxifying over 50 commonly used pharmaceutical drugs. Grapefruit juice is the best known of the inhibitors of this enzyme. Drinking grapefruit juice can greatly prolong the time caffeine will stay in your system, and if drunk too late at night, can result in severe insomnia if coffee has been consumed as well. Curcumin stimulates this enzyme, meaning it will reduce the time caffeine stays in your system.

Plant effects are even more complicated. Take, for example, cruciferous vegetables, such as broccoli. These plants contain a substance (sulforaphanes) that inhibits the CYP3A enzymes, but also contain indole-3-carbinol, which increases the enzyme's activity. In essence, one plant compound neutralizes the other.

Many plant flavonoids improve phase II function. Cruciferous vegetables for example, can enhance UDP-glucuronosyltrans-ferase activity, which is a critical phase II detoxification enzyme. Other foods that stimulate these beneficial enzymes include dandelion extract, rooibos and honeybush teas, pumpkin, carrots, squash, sweet potatoes, collards, red pepper, apples, onions, kale, cherries, red wine, extra virgin olive oil, beans, Brussels sprouts, broccoli, grapefruit, tomatoes, rosemary, ellagic acid, ferulic acid, curcumin, and astaxanthin. Magnesium-rich foods are also important for liver detoxification. These include halibut, almonds, cashews, spinach, oatmeal, peanuts, and wheat bran, in order of magnesium content. Keep in mind that the most important of our two systems for detoxification protection is the phase II system. This is the one that gets the toxic substances out of your body.

A long list of natural products has been shown to increase glutathione in the liver and other cells. These include curcumin, silymarin, folic acid, N-acetyl-L-cysteine (NAC), duck, egg yolks, cheese, red peppers, garlic, onions, and R-lipoic acid, among others. Glutathione itself is a powerful detoxification compound but also works as the special detoxification compound called *glutathione-S-transferase.*

Several foods increase the sulfur content needed for this type of detoxification. These include scallops, lobster, crab, peanuts, shrimp, veal, Brazil nuts, haddock, sardines, and eggs, in decreasing order.

While most attention has been paid to how foods either stimulate or inhibit these detoxification enzymes, more recent research has found that several natural products, rather than either stimulating or suppressing detoxification enzymes, will modulate these enzymes. This means they stimulate the enzymes if they are deficient and suppress them if they are overactive—the best of all worlds. Pomegranate, curcumin, cruciferous vegetables, green tea, and artichoke hearts seem to possess this modulation property, which is very valuable.

We should also keep in mind that many of the natural compounds are highly protective of the liver by a great number of mechanisms, beyond their effect on detoxification enzymes. For example, many are powerful antioxidants, anti-inflammatories, suppress cancer development, engage in antimicrobial activity (kill bacteria, viruses, and fungi), and increase the generation of factors that stimulate liver regeneration, such as sirtuins and bcl-2. Curcumin, quercetin, silymarin, and several of the carotenoids have these properties.

Special Liver Protectors

Curcumin

Curcumin, an extract of the spice turmeric, has demonstrated remarkable beneficial effects against a number of conditions, including cancer, brain disorders, prevention of the cytokine storm, reduction in autoimmune conditions, and liver protection. Curcumin has very powerful antioxidant and anti-inflammatory effects. It protects glutathione, potentiates the benefits of NAC, restores liver enzymes, inhibits lipid peroxidation, and most impressive of all, it stimulates the repair of a damaged liver. Curcumin is one of the more powerful stimulants for the production of the cell signaling factor called *sirtuins*, particularly sirt1. This factor plays a major role in liver regeneration. Turmeric contains only about 10 to 15% curcumin compounds. Unfortunately, curcumin is poorly absorbed as a pure compound. The Nano-Curcumin formulation (by One Planet Nutrition, Inc.) is very well absorbed and highly purified. Curcumin has a very high safety profile, but it is an iron chelator, so it should be given with vitamin C 30 minutes before a meal to prevent iron depletion.

Anthocyanins

This is a compound found abundantly in red wine, grapes, blueberries, blackberries, black currents, and red cabbage. Studies have shown this compound, and foods high in its content, can protect the liver from damage by chemicals, due to the compound's powerful antioxidant effects, by suppressing certain CYP-450 enzymes, and through a number of other mechanisms. Not only were liver enzymes such as AST improved, but actual histological repair was seen.

Apigenin

This is a flavonoid compound found in higher concentrations in celery, oranges, onions, parsley, and grapefruit and is also available as a supplement. In studies using mice, apigenin was shown to protect their livers from acetaminophen toxicity, stimulate the repair of liver tissue damage, reduce lipid peroxidation, and increase the content of glutathione in the liver. It also sooths and heals the lining of the intestines. It has very low toxicity.

Berberine

This is a compound isolated from a special plant, Berberis aristate, that has been shown to inhibit CYP-450 enzymes, thereby reducing conversion of procarcinogen chemicals into fully carcinogenic chemicals by the liver's phase I CYP-450 enzymes. Importantly, it has been shown to reduce fatty liver problems secondary to dietary deficiencies in choline and liver inflammation. Berberine uniquely inhibits the main inflammatory mechanism responsible for acetaminophen liver damage and damage by other drugs. It does this by inhibiting inflammasomes. Berberine also corrects insulin resistance and corrects type 2 diabetes in many cases.

Hesperidin

This is a flavonoid found in citrus fruits such as oranges, tangerines, and grapefruits. A number of studies have shown this flavonoid protects the liver by way of its powerful antioxidant effects, and its ability to restore antioxidant enzymes in the liver, reduce inflammation, and prevent liver cell death. Hesperidin has an excellent safety profile and can be purchased as a supplement.

Luteolin

This flavonoid is found in a number of plants and fruits and is especially high in content in sweet green peppers, green hot chili peppers, chicory greens, celery, pumpkins, and artichokes. Luteolin has potent antioxidant effects, anti-inflammatory effects, and has been shown to restore liver enzymes and replenish liver antioxidant enzymes. It also prevents glutathione from being depleted from the liver and restores damaged liver tissue. As an additional benefit, it has been shown to reduce brain fog.

Meso-Zeaxanthin

Meso-zeaxanthin is a carotenoid that plays a major role in protecting the macula of the eye. In addition, it has been shown to be very effective in protecting the liver by raising glutathione levels, restoring liver enzymes, acting as a powerful antioxidant, and repairing the liver cell damage caused by toxic chemicals, such as acetaminophen. It can be purchased as a supplement.

Pterostilbene

This compound is found in high concentrations in blueberries. After being absorbed from the GI tract, it is converted into resveratrol. It is far better absorbed than resveratrol and has a high degree of safety. Studies have shown that this compound has strong anti-inflammatory effects, is a powerful antioxidant,

protects the liver from acetaminophen toxicity, reduces lipid peroxidation, enhances liver antioxidant enzymes, inhibits inflammatory cytokines, and repairs liver cell damage. It can be purchased
as a supplement.

Schisandra

Compounds extracted from this plant have shown powerful liver
protective effects. A number of compounds have been isolated
from Schisandra, all of which are liver protective. Protection
arises from the plant's antioxidant effects, its inhibition of lipid
peroxidation, restoration of the liver's enzymes, reduction in some
of the CYP-450 enzymes, increased activation of the liver cells'
main antioxidant system (Nrf2), and by stimulating liver cell
repair. This compound can be purchased as a supplement and has
a good safety profile.

Silybin (Silymarin)

Most people have heard of silymarin and consider it to be the main
liver protecting natural compound. While it has demonstrated
impressive liver protective properties, it may not be as effective as
some of the other compounds listed earlier. It has been shown to
reduce lipid peroxidation, prevent glutathione depletion, and significantly reduce acetaminophen toxicity. It has a very good safety
profile and is useful for a great number of other health conditions,
especially prevention and treatment of various cancers, promoting prostate health, and protecting brain functions.

Zinc

Zinc is an essential element for health. Like many minerals, zinc intake should be controlled to prevent excess consumption. This is because excessive intakes can result in neurological injury, yet it takes substantially high doses to cause this damage. Many foods naturally have sufficiently high zinc levels for health, such as meats and most nuts.

The advantage of having sufficient zinc intake is that zinc stimulates the production of metallothionein, a compound found naturally in high levels in the cells lining the GI tract and in the liver itself. Metallothionein binds toxic metals such as lead, mercury, cadmium, copper, and arsenic. It usually takes about 3 weeks for zinc to increase metallothionein levels in tissues. Zinc also has antioxidant properties and is essential as a co-enzyme in a large number of biochemical reactions.

Excessive zinc intake can result in copper deficiency, which can manifest as headaches, increased sweating, transient elevation in some of the liver enzymes, and eventually sideroblastic anemia. To prevent this, I would recommend taking the zinc supplement every other day, and no more than 15 mg a day. Zinc comes in several forms. Zinc sulfate and zinc chloride are inexpensive, but can cause gastric upset.

The best absorbed and tolerated form of zinc is zinc acetate. You can supplement with low levels of copper, also an essential element, yet like iron and zinc, in higher levels of intake it is quite toxic to tissues and cells. The safe dose of copper for adults is no more than 3 mg a day. Copper infused water taken in limited amounts is a safe way to supplement with copper.

If a person has evidence of liver cirrhosis, they should not take copper supplements or eat foods high in copper, as they already have very high copper levels in their liver, which worsens the damage. Cirrhotics also have very low liver zinc levels, which aggravates the high copper levels. Zinc supplementation in such situations is beneficial.

Foods high in copper include chocolate, nuts, crustaceans (crab, lobster, etc.), and mushrooms.

Magnesium

Magnesium deficiency is very common with liver diseases, and universal with cirrhosis. Even worse, a deficiency in magnesium can worsen and accelerate the liver degeneration, for example, as seen in cirrhosis. Magnesium deficiency will significantly worsen inflammation in tissues of the liver and impairs the mitochondria's ability to produce energy, which also worsens free radical generation and lipid peroxidation, the primary processes causing liver damage.

Unfortunately, magnesium deficiency is quite common in this modern era, as people eat far less magnesium-containing foods, such as leafy green vegetables, nuts, pumpkin seeds, spinach, and tuna. Excessive consumption of alcohol dramatically lowers magnesium levels, as does stress and inflammation, especially chronic inflammation. Studies have shown that combining selenium (as selenomethionine) with magnesium produces even better liver protection against free radicals and lipid peroxidation.

CHAPTER 3

Did You Inherit
Your Liver Problem?

Anyone can develop liver disease—particularly given certain factors in our American lifestyle that include alcohol abuse, smoking, use of pharmaceutical drugs, illicit drug use, unhealthy foods, food additives, exposure to environmental toxic substances, and inactivity. However, there are also certain genetic factors that elevate risk.

In this chapter, I briefly discuss several diseases that can be inherited, or at least show a tendency to be inherited. If you have a family member with any of these diseases, you need to be especially vigilant. While these disorders are genetically inherited, one also needs to be aware of epigenetic influences. The best way to visualize epigenetics is to imagine that the various genes each have "on" and "off" switches. Things in the environment can either turn these switches "on" or "off." The "on" position activates the gene, whereas the "off" position shuts the gene down so it doesn't work—that is, it remains silent.

The field of epigenetics is growing rapidly as we begin to appreciate that many things can influence these gene switches throughout our lives. This can include industrial chemicals, pesticides, herbicides and fungicides, city pollution, household cleaners, various foods, food dyes, additives used in processed foods, vaccines, and a long list of other things. Due to their ability to affect these "on" and "off" gene switches, these epigenetic factors can have a major influence on the health of the liver and its ability to effectively detoxify harmful substances.

Researchers are finding that certain exposures to pollutants during fetal development can cause diseases to appear decades after a child is born. For example, being exposed to certain chemicals during life inside a baby's time in the womb can greatly increase a child's risk of developing Parkinson's disease during middle age. This has been found to be true for heart disease, liver disease, kidney disease, and especially brain disorders.

How Genetics Works

Before we get into liver diseases that are inheritable or otherwise genetically linked, let's talk about the science behind it.

The cells of our body contain genes that make up our DNA. This assortment of genes is known as the "genetic code." These genes, contained in 23 pairs of chromosomes, exercise a great deal of control over the baby's development, as well as cell function throughout the person's life. The genes mostly do this by controlling the creation of the many thousands of special proteins the cell uses for all its many functions and in maintaining its physical structure.

When the egg and sperm meet at the moment of conception, their individual chromosomes combine to create the new DNA code for the newly created life—the baby. Our DNA programs the cells for most of its functions, including when to multiply, and in many cases, when to die (called *apoptosis* or *programmed cell death*).

Some diseases are directly inherited, and some have a genetic predisposition, also called a *genetic susceptibility*. Having a genetic susceptibility to a disease means that possessing these particular genes, while not actually causing a disease, puts the person at a higher risk of developing the disease, especially if they are exposed to certain toxic substances. We call these "triggering" substances.

Some people with a predisposing genetic variation will never get the disease as long as they are not exposed to the particular toxic substance or stressful condition that acts as the final trigger. For example, if the harmful gene is triggered by exposure to a chemical used in the production of bricks, but you never come into contact with that chemical, you will never get the disease.

If you have a family member that has experienced a liver disease, be aware that you might be more vulnerable to the same or similar liver disorder. Because early treatment is important with most liver diseases, you should alert your doctor to a family history of such diseases, so you can undergo certain liver tests or, if indicated, genetic testing.

Also, if a liver disease runs in your family, you should avoid alcohol and other substances known to cause liver damage or stress on the liver.

Now let us look at some hereditary diseases known to affect the liver.

Celiac Disease

Celiac disease is a serious autoimmune disorder where the ingestion of gluten leads to damage in the small intestine and subsequent injury to many organs, including the liver and the brain. It is estimated to affect 1 in 100 people worldwide. Most cases go undiagnosed, with two and one-half million Americans being undiagnosed, and subsequently being at risk for long-term health complications, including liver damage.

When people with celiac disease eat gluten (a protein commonly found in wheat, rye, and barley), their body mounts an immune response that attacks the lining cells of the small intestine. These attacks lead to damage to the villi, small fingerlike projections that line the small intestine, that are mostly responsible for nutrient absorption. When the villi get damaged, nutrients cannot be absorbed properly into the body, resulting in deficiencies in a number of nutrients, including vitamins, proteins, carbohydrates, and fats. In severe cases of poor absorption, we call the condition **malabsorption**, which can result in severe weight loss and extreme vitamin deficiencies. Less severe cases of poor nutrient absorption can be quite difficult to diagnose, often taking decades before the problem is recognized. It is now thought that most cases begin during childhood and are not diagnosed until much later in life and sometimes never. These unrecognized cases result in a lifetime of poor health, constant fatigue, aching joints, and poor mental abilities (brain fog).

Foods high in gluten include wheat, rye, barley, spelt, and kamut (an ancient variety of wheat). While people with full-blown celiac disease have a genetic link, it is now known that everyone is sensitive to the harmful effects of gluten if consumed in high enough concentrations. The amount of gluten now being consumed is far greater than before special wheat products were engineered to contain such high gluten levels. If this were not bad enough, additional gluten is added to many processed foods, such as breads, cereals, and pastries. Between 1975 and the year 2000, gluten disease has increased some fivefold in the U.S. The highest incidence is among cases of type 1 diabetes, people with IgA deficiency, and those with Down syndrome.

The lowest incidence of celiac disease is found in sub-Saharan Africa and Japan, mainly because of the low consumption of gluten-containing foods and a low incidence of celiac-linked genes. The highest incidence is in the U.S.

The most common symptoms seen in severe cases of this disease included diarrhea alternating with constipation, abdominal cramping, muscle wasting, irritability, and sleep disturbances—almost all of which are related directly to the gastrointestinal tract. Poor absorption of fats can lead to severe depletion of fat-soluble vitamins, such as vitamins D, E, and K, and loose fat-filled stools.

Because it affects the intestinal cells, severe cases of the disease can cause impaired absorption of fats and proteins, and to a lesser extent carbohydrates. Victims of this disorder—called *malabsorption*—were also unable to absorb many vitamins and minerals critical for good health.

Celiac disease is not strictly genetically inherited, but it does tend to run in families. According to the Celiac Disease Foundation, people with a first-degree relative with celiac disease (parent, child, sibling) have a 1 in 10 risk of developing celiac disease. Individuals having the HLA-DQ2 or HLA-DQ8 genes are at the greatest risk. The incidence among identical twins is between 75 and 80%, far higher than just first-degree relatives (~10 to 15%). Individuals born homozygous (having both sets of mutated genes) for celiac disease not only have a much higher risk, somewhere around 25 to 30%, but also are more likely to have the condition appear during infancy.

As stated, not everyone with gluten sensitivity has a genetic link. That is, everyone is sensitive to gluten toxicity should they consume a high enough concentration of gluten in their diet, even if they have no celiac disease genes. The main problem is that gluten is not digestible by humans, and therefore when it leaks into the bloodstream from your GI tract, it acts as an immune antigen that mimics components in your tissues (called *molecular mimicry*). Because these components look so much alike, your immune system not only attacks the gluten but also any tissue that looks like gluten.

It should also be appreciated that gluten contains a compound called *gliadin*, which contains glutamate components that can also cause problems by triggering excitotoxicity. Gliadins can also cause the normally tight barrier of the intestinal lining (tight junctions) to break down, which allows these immune-stimulating food components to enter the blood stream. Keep in mind that the intestines have a special blood circulation that goes directly to the liver (hepatic portal system), which carries the gluten straight to the liver, where it can cause damage by inducing liver inflammation.

The intestinal damage occurs because some of the gluten and gliadin becomes trapped within the cells lining the intestine, mainly within the villi. The immune system attacks these trapped particles, destroying the villi. It has been theorized that some people fail to recover even after going on a gluten-free diet, because these trapped particles keep triggering an immune attack. It is important to keep in mind that 80% of the immune system resides in the wall of the intestines.

As with many conditions, we are finding that probiotic organisms are playing a major role in gluten sensitivity and celiac disease. Studies have shown that children with a family risk of celiac disease have fewer bacteroidetes-type organisms, and a higher concentration of firmicutes organisms in their colon than normal infants. Several probiotic organisms have been shown to protect against developing celiac disease.

Celiac disease is more common in women than men, with a ratio of 2:1 to 3:1, and can occur at any age. There are two major peaks: early childhood and the senior years. The disease is divided into a number of classifications, but suffice to say, the most important system breaks it into a predominantly **intestinal form** and an **extraintestinal form**.

The **intestinal** form mainly centers around GI problems, such as bloating, abdominal pain, diarrhea or alternating constipation/diarrhea, and in severe cases, extreme weight loss. In extreme cases, we see major malabsorption, nausea, chronic diarrhea, and occasional vomiting. Some 80% of children with celiac disease have no symptoms, which puts them at risk of a slow accumulation of damage to many organs over decades before they are eventually diagnosed.

Less recognized by most physicians is the **extraintestinal** (outside the intestine) form, which can mainly involve other organs, such as the liver, leading to anemia (malabsorption of vitamin B_{12} and folate), iron deficiency, osteoporosis, osteopenia, tooth enamel defects, and several neurological problems. In fact, the leading cause for cerebellar ataxia (a neurologic loss of balance) is celiac disease. One can also experience headaches, paresthesia (numbness), seizures, anxiety, and depression. This form is mostly seen in adults.

Reproductive problems can also occur with this disorder. A late onset of menarche (the onset of a woman's periods), amenorrhea (having no periods), recurrent miscarriages, premature birth of children, premature menopause, and, for men, a decrease in sperm count, are all associated with this disorder.

What has been called *subclinical celiac disease* is especially difficult to diagnose, if it is not suspected. In such cases, one can see a host of other autoimmune disorders, such as dermatitis herpetiformis, type I diabetes, Hashimoto's thyroiditis, selective IgA deficiency, alopecia areata, Addison's disease, hepatic autoimmune disorder, primary biliary cholangitis and primary sclerosing cholangitis (bile duct diseases), elevated liver enzymes, Sjögren's syndrome, and idiopathic dilated cardiomyopathy, a type of heart disease.

One of the most frightening links to this disorder is the high incidence of certain malignancies, such as non-Hodgkin's lymphoma, which is a type of cancer that starts in the white blood cells. In fact, in prolonged celiac disease, one sees a six- to nine-fold increased risk in this malignancy. The highest incidence of this ailment is in people with celiac disease who do not respond to a gluten-free diet. That is, despite avoiding all gluten in their diet, their symptoms continue, a condition we call **refractory celiac disease**. Individuals with this form of celiac disease have a 33% to 52% increased risk of developing a malignancy within the next 5 years after diagnosis.

Several medical studies have linked fatty liver disease with celiac disease. In the largest and most recent study, published in June 2015 in the *Journal of Hepatology*, researchers compared the risk of developing nonalcoholic fatty liver disease in nearly 27,000 people with celiac disease to the risk in similar individuals without celiac.

The study found the risk of developing fatty liver disease to be nearly three times higher in those with celiac disease. Surprisingly, children with celiac had the highest risk of fatty liver disease. The risk of developing the liver condition was much higher in the first year following a celiac diagnosis but remained "significantly elevated" even 15 years beyond the celiac diagnosis.

In another 2011 study, which took place in Iran, researchers found celiac disease in 2.2% of patients with nonalcoholic fatty liver disease, most of whom were not overweight or obese. They concluded that clinicians should consider screening for celiac disease in people with fatty liver disease who don't have obvious risk factors for that condition, such as being overweight or obese.

Nonalcoholic fatty liver disease, a serious liver ailment currently on the rise in the U.S., is discussed further in Chapter 13.

While celiac disease is a much more serious disease, recent studies suggest that gluten sensitivity or gluten intolerance is much more common. In fact, it may affect up to 30 to 40% of the American population. As noted earlier, research has demonstrated that everyone is sensitive to gluten if enough is ingested with meals, and with food manufacturers adding more and more gluten to foods, the problem can only get worse.

Symptoms of non-celiac gluten sensitivity are similar to those of celiac disease and include stomach pain, bloating, changes in bowel movements, fatigue, brain fog, and eczema or a rash.

We have also learned that gluten sensitivity is a multisystem disease affecting a great number of systems in the body, along with the GI tract. For example, it affects fat metabolism, is associated with diabetes, can trigger autoimmune diseases (such as rheumatoid arthritis, lupus, and thyroid autoimmune disorders), and can affect the brain, including higher functions such as memory, learning, attention, and behavior. Considerable evidence suggests that a leading cause for schizophrenia is gluten intolerance, and that when gluten is removed from their diets, most will recover.

Testing for Gluten Sensitivity

The most accurate way to diagnose celiac disease is to take a biopsy of the duodenal mucosa, which shows atrophy of the villi—the finger-like microscopic projections on the surface of the duodenum. Laboratory tests also have a high degree of accuracy. The most commonly used blood tests include:

- Anti-tTG antibodies
- Anti-endomysium antibodies (EmA)
- Deaminated gliadin peptide antibodies (DGP)

Gastroenterologists use what is referred to as the "4 out of 5 rule" to make a definite diagnosis of celiac disease. That is, the person should have four of the five most common findings to be considered as having the disease:

- Typical signs and symptoms
- Serum antibody positive
- Have HLA-DQ2 or HLA-DQ8 positive genetic test
- Intestinal damage (demonstrated by biopsy)
- Clinical response to a gluten-free diet

Normally the tTG antibody test will revert to normal in 6 to 12 months of being on a gluten-free diet—but not in everyone. In highly sensitive people, even a very small amount of gluten in the diet can cause the onset of severe symptoms. Keep in mind that sometimes the gluten or gliadin (a peptide in the gluten cells) gets trapped in the cells lining the intestine, which can make symptoms persist and even progress. The longer a person goes undiagnosed, the more likely they will suffer serious consequences and even death.

Treatment

The only treatment accepted for celiac disease is to follow a gluten-free diet—that is, to avoid all foods that contain gluten. For most people, following this diet will stop symptoms, heal existing intestinal damage, and prevent further damage. Improvements begin within weeks of starting the diet. A gluten-free diet will also help alleviate symptoms in people with gluten sensitivity.

It was hoped that a set of digestive enzymes a person could take with each meal that would digest the normally indigestible gluten could be developed, but so far, the results have not been as impressive as with total avoidance of gluten.

While one may not be able to totally prevent gluten damage, the evidence suggests that the damage being done by the inflammation induced by the abnormal immune reaction can be reduced or even controlled. This means that things that reduce the immune reaction, such as increasing one's intake of omega-3 oils and avoiding the inflammatory omega-6 oils, sugar, and high-protein diets would help. Natural compounds, such as Nano-Curcumin, Nano-Grape Seed extract, Nano-Boswellia, and Nano-Quercetin would also reduce the immune overreaction and greatly reduce inflammation. All these compounds are highly absorbed, and in addition have powerful anticancer effects. The nano products can be found at the One Planet Nutrition Company website (www.oneplanetnutrition.com).

Hemochromatosis

Iron is essential for life, yet an excessive amount of iron when deposited in tissues and organs can be quite harmful and even lead to some deadly diseases, such as cancer, neurodegenerative diseases, diabetes, and liver failure.

Iron is essential for the following functions:

- Mitochondrial energy production (cellular energy)
- Muscle oxygenation (used by myoglobin in muscles)
- Production of antioxidant compounds (catalase)
- DNA replication and repair
- Immune function

The main disorder associated with excess iron is called **hemochromatosis**, a genetic condition associated with excessively high absorption and distribution of iron throughout the body, primarily in the liver, pancreas, heart, joints, and pituitary gland. This excess iron can cause liver cirrhosis, liver cancer, diabetes, and/or cardiomyopathy (heart failure), possibly resulting in death.

The most dangerous iron is free iron or unbound iron. Normally, the majority of iron is bound to special proteins, such as **transferrin** and **ferritin**, designed to protect tissues from iron damage. A certain amount of iron is not bound, and we call this free iron. Unbound iron can trigger the intense generation of some very harmful free radicals.

Free radicals are generated by the metabolic process and, as we age, more of this inflammation is produced, and the body accumulates more iron than is safe. This results in our bodies becoming more inflamed, which increases tissue aging and organ damage, especially brain damage. Men accumulate iron earlier than women. Women periodically lose iron during menstruation. After menopause, women accumulate iron faster than men.

Iron accumulation increases free radical formation and lipid peroxidation (oxidation of fats in our tissues)—a very dangerous situation. Iron accumulation can cause increased damage in cases of multiple sclerosis, strokes, heart attacks, trauma, Parkinson's disease, and Alzheimer's disease, and it significantly worsens infectious diseases, including viral diseases. It is known that giving iron during a serious active infection can kill a patient because the bacteria use the iron to multiply. In fact, during infections, the body normally will reduce the amount of available iron in the body, in an effort to starve the bacteria. Chronic inflammatory diseases, such as rheumatoid arthritis, are associated with very low iron levels in the blood. As a result, anemia is very common with chronic inflammatory diseases. Raising iron levels in these patients helps in some ways, but can also worsen the inflammation.

Iron is also a powerful stimulus for cancer growth and its spread, and for invasion of the cancer into surrounding healthy cells—in fact, I consider it to be a cancer fertilizer. Iron stimulates cancer growth for the very same reason it worsens infections—it stimulates cell reproduction. Some advanced cancer treatments utilizing methods to lower tissue iron levels have shown impressive results.

Mutation in the HFE gene, which controls iron metabolism, is not expressed completely until both genes, one donated by each parent, is present—called **homozygosis gene expression**. There is some evidence that people inheriting only one gene (**heterozygotes**) can also have iron metabolism abnormalities, just not as obvious as the homozygous gene carriers. Yet, several studies have shown that having only one of these hemochromatosis genes can cause some serious health problems.

For example, studies have shown that even having mild iron excess, as seen with heterozygotes, can increase one's susceptibility to nonalcoholic fatty liver disease (NAFLD), is associated with greater liver fibrosis in cases of hepatitis C infection, is associated with a greater incidence of cardiovascular death in women, and a significantly greater risk of certain cancers, such as colon cancer, gastric cancer, liver cancer, and breast cancer. One study found that having slightly elevated iron levels increased one's risk of damage by radiation, which would be especially important in women having yearly breast mammograms, especially because the breast is one of the most sensitive tissues in the body to induction of cancer by radiation exposure. MRI scanning of the breast is far safer and more accurate.

Normally, iron absorption is very tightly controlled. Even though the usual diet contains 20 mg of iron, we absorb only 1 to 2 mgs per day. Most iron is absorbed in the upper small intestine (duodenum). With the condition hemochromatosis, a great deal more iron is absorbed. One of the areas in the body most affected by high iron levels is the brain. Studies have shown that people with hemochromatosis are at a fivefold higher risk of developing Alzheimer's disease.

One of the first events in the development of Parkinson's disease, long before symptoms develop, is an abnormal accumulation of excess iron in the part of the brain most affected (substantia nigra). In both cases, the excess iron is causing inflammation, free radical accumulation, and lipid peroxidation in the brain—a very damaging combination. And in both of these conditions, it is free iron that is most harmful. Free iron excess is also linked to the dramatic increase in cardiovascular disease seen with hemochromatosis. Zinc appears to protect against the iron toxicity seen in heart disease.

High levels of iron also play a major role in atherosclerosis, the process that causes increased heart attacks, strokes, and peripheral vascular disease. In fact, studies have shown that atherosclerotic plaque (arterial crud) contains high levels of free iron. Lowering iron reduces one's risk of these disorders. High iron levels raise blood cholesterol levels. Free iron also stimulates nitric oxide generation, which can combine with the free radical superoxide to form the very destructive radical **peroxynitrite**— which commonly occurs in the liver, kidneys, and other organs with iron toxicity.

Hemochromatosis occurs most commonly in Caucasians of Northern European descent, and symptoms usually occur after age 50, when significant iron has accumulated in the body. It is generally diagnosed in women about 10 years later, because, before menopause, women lose iron monthly due to menstruation. (There is a secondary form of the disease that can be caused by other ailments such as liver disease, anemia, blood transfusions, or thalassemia, another genetic disease.) Men are more likely to present with liver disease, and women with fatigue, arthritis, and excessive skin pigmentation.

The rate of iron accumulation and the subsequent appearance of symptoms, and their severity, varies widely from case to case. The most common early complaints include:

- Fatigue
- Weakness
- Joint pain
- Palpitations of the heart
- Abdominal pains

Much later in the course of the disease one may see:

- Hyperpigmented skin (bronzing of skin)
- Arthritis
- Liver cirrhosis
- Diabetes
- Severe fatigue
- Low reproductive hormone levels
- Hypopituitarism
- Enlarged heart (cardiomyopathy)
- Primary liver cancer
- Increased risk of bacterial infections

Abdominal pains are common in cases having cirrhosis. Hepatocellular carcinoma (liver cancer) is 200 times more common with hemochromatosis when associated with cirrhosis, and accounts for 30 to 45% of deaths of patients seen in referral centers.

Diabetes is also strongly associated with hemochromatosis. All symptoms worsen with aging, and iron accumulation accelerates the aging of all tissue and organs.

Hemochromatosis Treatment

The treatment of hemochromatosis involves the following:

- Avoiding iron supplements and foods high in iron levels
- Avoiding substances that damage the liver, such as alcohol abuse, smoking, MSG exposure, liver damaging drugs, and liver toxic sweeteners (aspartame and saccharine)
- Avoiding vitamin C supplements, especially with meals

The primary medical treatment is phlebotomy—periodic removal of blood. In most cases, this works very well. Fortunately, there are a number of natural compounds that are iron binding compounds (chelators), which can remove a great deal of the iron. The most important include:

- IP6 (phytic acid)
- Myoinositol
- Baicalin
- Nano-Curcumin
- Nano-Quercetin
- Nano-Grape Seed extract
- Silymarin
- Berberine
- Hesperidin
- Luteolin

The three most impressive of these natural compounds in reducing iron damage include IP6, hesperidin, and baicalin, which can be used in combination. Hesperidin, a flavonoid from citrus fruits, significantly reduces iron blood levels, prevents cellular damage by iron in the liver and kidneys, and restores normal functioning in these organs. Hesperidin is very safe to take even in larger doses.

Wilson's Disease

Wilson's disease is a rare genetic disorder, occurring in about one out of every 30,000 people. Both men and women are affected similarly.

This is a disease that causes an accumulation of excess copper in the body. We all have copper in our bodies, but in people with Wilson's disease, the copper isn't eliminated properly and instead accumulates in tissues, particularly in the liver, brain, and the corneas of the eyes. It is a progressive disease, and if untreated, can result in liver disease, central nervous system dysfunction, and death. But early diagnosis and treatment can help prevent these problems.

The high copper levels in the liver in this disease are associated with significant damage to liver cells (hepatocytes) and are associated with a high incidence of cirrhosis. Over time, this also increases the risk of developing liver cancer (hepatocarcinoma).

Damage from this disease can begin in childhood, but it usually manifests symptoms in people who are in their teenage years and early twenties. Common signs of associated liver disease include a yellow discoloration (jaundice) of the skin and the rim of the cornea of the eyes, as well as swelling of the legs and abdomen due to fluid retention, a tendency for bruising, prolonged bleeding, and fatigue. Some individuals with this disease may only show abnormalities on liver function tests and no symptoms until many years later.

As the disease progresses, it may cause neurological problems, some beginning when people are in their thirties. These can include tremors, involuntary movements, difficulty swallowing, lack of coordination, spasticity, dystonic postures (movement disorders), and muscle rigidity.

Almost all people with Wilson's disorder have characteristic rings at the rim of their eyes' corneas, called Kayser-Fleischer rings.

People with Wilso's disease can be treated. Treatment includes medications that prompt the organs to release copper into the bloodstream, from which it can be eliminated from the body. Zinc reduces the toxicity of copper and helps balance copper levels in the liver. Several flavonoids also chelate copper and can reduce, to some extent, the toxic effect of excess copper in the liver and other tissues. The most powerful copper chelators and compounds that reduce copper toxicity include Nano-EGCG, Nano-Curcumin, luteolin, Nano-Quercetin, and resveratrol. The most beneficial appears to be Nano-Curcumin.

Are You at Genetic Risk for Alcoholism and Alcoholic Liver Disease?

Inheriting a genetic disease is not the only way genetics can affect your liver. There is a growing body of evidence that the propensity to develop alcoholism may be genetically based.

Genetics can also affect how your body processes alcohol, or whether you are prone to developing alcoholism, which is the inability to control drinking due to both a physical and emotional dependence on alcohol. Other factors, such as environment, play a role, but there is abundant evidence indicating that alcoholism is a complex genetic disease, with variations in a large number of genes affecting risk. Some of these genes have been identified, including two genes of alcohol metabolism, ADH1B and ALDH2, that have the strongest impact on the risk for alcoholism. Of more importance are genes that are related to the complications and incidence of complications of alcoholism, such as simple fatty liver (steatosis), fatty liver with severe inflammation (steatohepatitis), liver fibrosis (scarring), liver cirrhosis, and hepatocellular carcinoma (liver cancer).

While fatty liver disease that is related to alcohol use is similar to nonalcoholic fatty liver disease (NAFLD), the former is associated with greater infiltration of the liver's lobules with inflammatory cells (neutrophils and macrophages), greater liver inflammation, and obvious necrosis of liver cells (death of these cells).

Alcoholism is considered to be a familial disorder, with a greater involvement of male than female family members (50% versus 22%). A careful study of twins found that alcohol abuse was 50% heritable and the rest is due to exposure to similar environmental factors.

Several genetic alterations (SNPs) have been linked to alcohol-related liver disease. One of the more commonly expressed is the **PNPLA3 gene**, which is a major risk factor for chronic liver disease progression—that is, a more rapid progression from a simple fatty liver to steatohepatitis, fibrosis, cirrhosis, and eventually hepatocellular carcinoma (liver cancer). The gene designated **TM6SF2** has been associated with the development of nonalcoholic fatty liver disease and its progression to worse liver damage as well. The third identified gene linked to liver disease promoted by alcohol consumption is designated **MBOAT7/TMC4**. People possessing this gene have a higher risk of developing cirrhosis when they are exposed to regular alcohol use.

It is known that Hispanic men (especially of Mexican origin) have the highest risk of developing alcohol-related liver cirrhosis, and they do so at a younger age. The PNPLA3 gene is more common among Hispanics. It is significantly less common among Caucasians and blacks, which would account for the finding that these ethnic groups have significantly less alcohol-induced liver fat accumulation and eventual cirrhosis.

The risk of developing liver cancer (hepatocarcinoma) is also higher in those carrying the PNPLA3 gene. In addition, alcoholic patients with liver cirrhosis carrying the TM6SF2 gene are also at a higher risk of this liver cancer. Having both the PNPLA3 gene and the TM6SF2 gene accounts for half of all cases of hepato-carcinoma. If this is not bad enough, having the MBOAT7 gene increases the risk of developing liver cancer by 80% in Italian men with cirrhosis and even increases the risk in men without cirrhosis.

There are several other gene mutations associated with an increased risk of liver disease among alcoholics, most involve pro-tective mechanisms that normally would protect the liver, but in these individuals these mechanisms are defective. Most important are the antioxidant enzymes, as most of the liver damage is caused by high levels of free radicals and lipid peroxidation products.

Epigenetic Mechanisms

As I mentioned earlier, genes are controlled by what can be thought of as "on" and "off" switches. The "on" switch activates the gene so it becomes fully operational. The "off" switch silences the gene, so it does not work. Operation of these switches is what we call epigenetics—that is, various outside influences can operate these gene "switches." For example, alcohol, pesticides, herbicides, fungicides, stress, hormones, dietary factors, food additives, and a host of other things can operate these switches.

In the case of liver diseases, the effect of turning these switches "on" and "off" can mean the induction of many factors, or the silencing of these same factors. The most common ultimate epi-genetic controls by which these "switches" do their job is by three main mechanisms—DNA methylation, histone modifications, and RNA silencing (via microRNAs)—all of which control DNA function. As an example of how alcohol can affect these mechanisms, research shows that alcohol can regulate microR-NAs (miRNA), and these miRNAs control various genes related to liver health.

It is also important to understand that these epigenetic "switches," especially the sensitivity and control of these switches, can be inherited. A person inheriting a "weakness" for a particular epigenetic switch control would be at a greater risk of liver problems should they drink alcohol.

Important in the pathology of alcoholic liver diseases is immune activation and subsequent liver inflammation—which is chronic, as long as a person abuses alcohol. The combined toxicity of the alcohol on liver cells and chronic activation of the liver's immune cells (especially macrophages) results in progressive and quite severe liver damage. Stopping the alcohol consumption before irreversible cirrhosis or liver cancer develops can reverse much of the damage, especially if one supplements with liver nutrients, vitamins, and minerals.

Inflammation within the liver causes the generation of massive numbers of free radicals and lipid peroxidation products (called *oxidative damage*), which can destroy liver cells and severely impair the function of the cells that survive. Things that reduce this oxidative damage, promote liver regeneration, and switch on genes that are protective can reverse a great deal of this damage and even protect against such damage occurring in the first place.

Nano-Curcumin, Nano-Quercetin, Nano-Silymarin, hesperidin, taurine, vitamin E (especially mixed tocotrienols), B-complex vitamins, selenium (as selenomethionine), sulfur-containing foods, and pterostilbene all protect the liver and promote liver regeneration. They also reduce liver immune overactivation.

CHAPTER 4

Liver Symptoms and Tests

Your liver is a remarkable organ that plays a huge number of roles in your body.

The goal of this book is to show you how to keep your liver healthy, but there are many threats your liver faces, and these range from your external environment to things you may knowingly or unknowingly ingest, as well as viruses or other diseases over which you have no control.

The result is that a variety of liver diseases can occur. Some have their own symptoms, and diagnostic tests associated with them, which are discussed in later chapters.

Many liver diseases and disorders, however, have certain symptoms in common, and there are general tests that can be used to diagnose them. It is these that are discussed in this chapter.

What Type of Doctor Should You See?

The doctor who provides your general medical care will probably be the first you see for a possible liver problem. We'll call this your primary care physician (PCP) even though they may be an internist or family doctor. But the point is that, unless you have a very common problem, it is likely that, after your diagnosis, you will be referred to a specialist, such as a gastroenterologist or hepatologist.

Even if that's the case, you'll want to keep your PCP involved as part of your health care team. Your PCP can help you make informed decisions about your care and will also serve as a liaison among your other doctors. Also, many diseases have a lifestyle component; for instance, you may need to lose weight if you are diagnosed with nonalcoholic fatty liver disease, or reduce your alcohol intake if you have cirrhosis, and your PCP can help guide you in making needed lifestyle changes, or refer you to substance abuse or mental health specialists, or a naturopath if you need them.

Here are the specialists you may be referred to:

Gastroenterologist

A gastroenterologist is a doctor who is board certified in internal medicine, as well as gastroenterology. In order to obtain this certification, the doctor must have completed a two- to three-year fellowship in gastroenterology, which involves studying disorders of the digestive tract, including the liver, stomach, intestines, pancreas, and gallbladder.

Hepatologist

A hepatologist is trained specifically to treat disorders of the liver, as well as its associated organs: the pancreas and gallbladder. Although no specific board certification goes along with this specialty, the doctor must complete a one- to two-year fellowship in a broad area of liver diseases.

Both gastroenterologists and hepatologists are trained in treating diseases of the liver.

Other Types of Specialists

If you have an infectious disease, such as HIV along with hepatitis, your team may include an infectious disease specialist. If liver cancer is your problem, you may also see an oncologist, who is a doctor that specializes in cancer, in addition to either a gastroenterologist or a hepatologist. One can also work with natural physicians specializing in the treatment of cancer.

No matter which type of doctor you decide upon, remember that it is up to you to decide on whether you feel a certain level of mutual trust, openness, and attentiveness.

Five Questions to Ask a Prospective Doctor

In addition to asking whether your prospective doctor takes your insurance and what their office policies are, you'll want to ask about their training and expertise. Here are some suggested questions:

- What specific training do you have in liver diseases?
- What percentage of your practice is devoted to patients with liver diseases?
- Do you keep abreast of new and experimental treatments, and also clinical studies?
- Will I be seeing you or another doctor? (This can be an important question for doctors who are affiliated with medical schools.)
- What is your viewpoint on alternative and complementary medical treatments? (Even if you are primarily interested in conventional or Western medical treatment, it may be important to you that your doctor can at least listen to such alternative viewpoints with an open mind.)

Signs and Symptoms of Liver Disease

One of the problems with liver disease is that by the time you are diagnosed, the ailment is advanced, and significant damage to the liver has already been done. Although the liver does have a remarkable ability to regenerate, this cannot occur if too much healthy tissue is lost, says Dr. Anrug Maheshwari, a gastroenterologist who specializes in liver disorders for Mercy Medical Center's Institute for Digestive Health and Liver Disease in Baltimore.

Because liver disease doesn't cause any symptoms until it's advanced, it's too often overlooked by patients—and sometimes their doctors as well.

"One of the things that we have struggled with is a proactive approach to dealing with liver disease and getting people motivated to act sooner and earlier in terms of being able to prevent serious complications," he says.

In the case of many liver diseases, the first and only symptom may be jaundice. The vast majority of the other symptoms discussed here generally only become apparent when liver disease is quite advanced, which is why it's important to catch liver disease early, before problems like scarring and severe liver damage occur.

This is an important reason why, if you think you may have a liver disease, you need to make sure your doctor takes your concerns seriously.

Liver Disease Symptoms

Jaundice

Skin and eyes that appear yellowish is from a condition known as jaundice. Jaundice forms when there is too much bilirubin in your system. Bilirubin is a yellow pigment that is created by the breakdown of dead red blood cells in the liver. Normally, the liver gets rid of bilirubin along with old red blood cells. Since most liver diseases don't have early symptoms, jaundice may be the first that appears, so if this happens to you, make sure you take your concerns to your doctor promptly. Jaundice usually indicates obstruction of the liver drainage system, such as intrahepatic channels or bile ducts.

Pain

A dull aching in the right area of the abdomen, just below the ribs. This can indicate liver pain, which can be the result of a variety of causes, including ascites (fluid in the abdomen), cirrhosis, hepatitis, liver failure, a liver abscess, and liver cancer. Gas trapped in the right hepatic flexure of the colon can cause a similar pain, especially in people with the irritable colon disorder, as this part of the colon is adjacent to the liver.

Weight Loss

Unexplained weight loss or loss of appetite can be a symptom of advanced liver disease.

Abdominal Pain and Swelling

A swollen abdomen can point to a condition called *ascites*, which can occur when there is a liver malfunction that has resulted in an imbalance of proteins and other compounds. It also occurs with obstruction of the hepatic veins. This can occur due to advanced cirrhosis.

Swelling

Swelling in the legs and ankles can be another sign of advanced liver damage due to cirrhosis and often accompanies ascites.

Itchy Skin

Liver disease can result in the accumulation of bile salts under the skin, which can result in severe itching.

Dark Urine

Urine can turn dark because of the bilirubin excreted through the kidneys. High levels of bilirubin may be attributed to inflammation, or other abnormalities of the liver cells, or blockage of the bile ducts. Bilirubin is an orange-yellow pigment formed in the liver by the breakdown of red blood cells. It is excreted through bile.

Unusual Colored Stool

Pale stool color, or bloody or tar-colored stool: If the stools are pale, it may indicate a problem with the liver or other part of the biliary drainage system. Stool that floats and is light colored or very pale indicates a deficiency of the necessary bile needed for fat absorption. This can result from bile duct obstruction or other liver problems. Black tarry stools can happen in advanced liver disease and are caused by blood passing through the gastrointestinal tract. This can indicate a medical emergency.

Chronic Fatigue

Extreme tiredness, exhaustion, and fatigue is a symptom of advanced liver disease, although its cause is a matter of debate. Some experts believe it is due to changes in brain chemistry resulting from impaired liver function; others believe it is because of a buildup of toxins, or altered levels of hormones that may be at the root of low energy levels.

Nausea or Vomiting

This is another sign of advanced liver disease as the body becomes unable to process and eliminate toxins. The tendency to bruise easily is another sign of advanced liver disease because it indicates that the liver is no longer functioning properly and has lost its ability to produce proteins enabling the blood to clot.

The Stages of Liver Disease

There are many types of liver disease, which are different in many ways, but they do have some things in common. One of these is that many, but not all, liver diseases tend to go through different stages, during which the organ becomes further and further compromised.

No matter which liver disease you have—whether your liver has been damaged by a virus, chemicals, an immune disease, alcohol, or other condition—the basic danger is the same: The liver will become so damaged that it will no longer be able to perform its functions.

The following is an example of the stages the liver can pass through. As you'll see, interrupting this disease process at an early stage can help the liver regain its functioning and stop the downward slide.

The Healthy Liver

A healthy liver is not diseased and is capable of performing all of its lifesaving functions, including digesting food, storing energy compounds (glycogen), storing oil-soluble vitamins, and protecting your body from poisons. It can also regenerate itself, which means it can grow back if it is damaged.

Inflammation

The earliest sign of liver disease is when the organ becomes inflamed. This is a signal that it has been injured, but is trying to heal. You commonly see this if you cut your finger; the area of the injury becomes reddened and painful. That it has become inflamed is obvious. The problem with liver inflammation is that it is often a chronic low-grade, smoldering inflammation, which means that it occurs deep in the body, is invisible, and if nothing interrupts the inflammation process, the damage to the liver will persist and worsen.

Fibrosis

If inflammation goes unchecked, the inflamed liver begins to scar. This means that scarred tissue replaces healthy liver tissue, a process known as fibrosis. Scarred tissue cannot provide the functions that healthy liver tissue can. Even worse, scarred tissue can build up, and the result is that this can obstruct the flow of blood and hepatic channels within the liver, causing further damage.

Cirrhosis

Cirrhosis is what happens when hard, scarred tissue replaces soft, healthy liver tissue. As cirrhosis becomes worse, the amount of healthy tissue in the liver diminishes, and if cirrhosis is not treated, the liver will eventually fail. Cirrhosis can also lead to liver cancer. Once you've been diagnosed with cirrhosis, treatment will center on trying to slow the cirrhosis process and protect the healthy liver tissue that's left.

End-Stage Liver Disease

This includes a subgroup of people with cirrhosis that have symptoms, including many discussed earlier, that are untreatable. This stage may also be known as liver failure. At this stage a liver transplant is the only option.

Liver Disease Diagnostic Tests

Blood Tests

Liver Function Panel

There is no one specific test to check on how well the liver is functioning, so several different tests are done that comprise what is called the *liver function panel*, or the *hepatic function panel*.

This test uses specific readings to measure the levels of total protein, albumin, bilirubin, and liver enzymes present in your blood. Levels that are too high or too low may indicate liver damage or disease.

This panel is part of the lab tests given during a general physical, which is good because it can act as a screening test for liver problems in people who are generally healthy.

On the other hand, general health care professionals don't interpret them as stringently as they should, and sometimes are too inclined to brush aside test results that show elevated liver enzymes, says Dr. Maheshwari.

Common reasons for elevated liver enzymes include:

- Over-the-counter drugs, particularly pain medications such as acetaminophen (Tylenol, etc.)
- Certain prescription medications, including cholesterol-lowering statin drugs

- Drinking alcohol
- Hepatitis A, B, and C
- Nonalcoholic fatty liver disease
- Obesity

Less common causes include the following:

- Alcoholic hepatitis (liver inflammation caused by alcohol)
- Autoimmune hepatitis (liver inflammation caused by an autoimmune disease such as celiac disease, rheumatoid arthritis, or hyperthyroidism (Grave's disease or Hashimoto's thyroiditis)
- Cytomegalovirus (a common virus that may cause no problems except in women who are pregnant or people with weakened immune systems)
- Epstein–Barr virus
- Hemochromatosis (too much iron stored in the body)
- Liver cancer
- Mononucleosis
- Polymyositis (an uncommon inflammatory disease that causes weakness)
- Sepsis
- Thyroid disorders
- Wilson's disease (too much copper stored in the body)

Liver Tests Too Often Ignored

But there is a problem with the liver function test. It isn't that it's not useful—it's a battery of very valuable tests. The problem is that doctors sometimes brush off abnormal results. That is why you should always get a copy of your lab tests, and if you notice any findings that are outside the "normal" level, carefully question your doctor about it. If an abnormal test result appears, have the test repeated in a couple of weeks to see if the results have returned to normal or are rising. Progressive elevation of these tests is a sign of significant disease.

In addition to being part of a regular lab screen, a liver function test is often recommended in the following situations:

- To monitor side effects if you're taking a medication that is known to affect the liver
- To check for damage from liver infections, such as hepatitis B and hepatitis C
- To check for a reason for the symptoms
- To monitor people at risk for liver problems if, for instance, they have high triglycerides, diabetes, high blood pressure, or have gallbladder disease or anemia
- To monitor heavy alcohol drinkers

What a Liver Function Test Measures

Protein

Protein is an essential nutrient made up of chemicals called *amino acids*, and is necessary for energy, fluid balance, and for maintaining and rebuilding all tissues and supporting the immune system. Your doctor will be checking to make sure there is enough protein in your blood to support your liver's functions.

Albumin

Albumin is a specific protein produced in the liver that helps prevent blood from leaking out of blood vessels, carries medicine and other substances through the blood, and is important for healing.

Bilirubin

Bilirubin is a substance produced when old red blood cells and hemoglobin, the protein in red blood cells, break down. Normally, the amount of bilirubin in the blood should be very low. If it's too high, it can cause the jaundiced color indicative of liver disease.

Ammonia

If the liver is not functioning properly, ammonia can build up. Ammonia is toxic to the brain.

Enzymes

Enzymes are produced by the body to speed up chemical reactions, such as energy metabolism, digestion, detoxification, and blood clotting. Abnormal enzyme levels can help diagnose certain liver problems. These include:

Alkaline Phosphatase

This test measures the enzyme alkaline phosphatase, or ALP. ALP is manufactured mostly in the liver and bone, with some made in the intestines and kidneys. A too-high level can indicate bone disease, such as Paget's disease, or cancer that has spread to the bone, vitamin D deficiency, damaged liver cells, or show that bile flow is blocked.

Aspartate Aminotransferase (AST)

This enzyme is normally found in red blood cells, liver, heart muscle tissue, the pancreas, and kidneys. Normally, the level is low; a too-high level can indicate heart or liver damage.

Alanine Aminotransferase (ALT)

ALT is another enzyme found mainly in the liver, although there are smaller amounts in the kidneys, heart, muscle, and pancreas. This is another test that can indicate liver damage.

International Normalized Ratio Test

The international normalized ratio test, or INR, is a blood test that evaluates the manner in which the blood clots. In the case of serious disease, especially cirrhosis, the liver may not produce the proper amount of proteins, and thus the blood will not able to clot as it should.

Hepatitis Tests

If hepatitis is suspected, your doctor can perform a blood test that will detect certain antibodies in your blood. These antibodies can show whether you have the hepatitis virus, and which type it is—hepatitis A, B, C, D, or E. In addition, the doctor performs a liver function test to find out if the hepatitis virus has caused any liver damage.

Blood Clotting Tests

The liver is responsible for blood clotting. Two tests can be performed to look at the organ's blood clotting functionality.

- **Partial thromboplastin time (PTT).** This test is done to check for blood clotting problems.
- **Prothrombin time (PT).** This test is commonly done to determine if a person is on the correct dose of the blood

thinner warfarin (Coumadin). It also can detect blood
clotting problems.

Imaging Tests

- **Abdominal ultrasound.** This is a non-invasive test done to
  detect many liver conditions, including cancer, cirrhosis, or
  gallstones.
- **MRI scan (computed technology).** An MRI scan can
  give more detailed images of the liver and other abdominal organs. For instance, an MRI scan of the liver and
  biliary tract can evaluate the liver, gallbladder, or their
  related structures for tumors, injuries, bleeding, infections,
  abscesses, obstructions, or other conditions. It is safer than
  a CT scan in that the MRI does not use radiation.

Liver Biopsy

- **Liver biopsy.** For a liver biopsy, a small needle is inserted
  into the liver to collect a sample of tissue, which is then
  analyzed. A liver biopsy is usually performed to diagnose
  a variety of diseases and disorders. For example, it can be
  done to identify the cause of persistent abnormal liver
  enzymes, unexplained jaundice (yellowing of the skin), a
  liver abnormality found on non-invasive tests like an ultrasound or CT scan, or unexplained liver enlargement.
- **Liver and spleen scan.** This test uses a small amount of
  radioactive material, called a *radionuclide*, to take pictures
  of your liver. A special device, called a *gamma camera*,
  provides images to show how well your liver and spleen
  are functioning. The spleen, which is involved in the

production and removal of blood cells, works closely with the liver. This test can detect liver cancer, nonmalignant cysts, abscesses, hematomas (bruise-like injuries), cirrhosis, and hepatitis, or monitor whether liver disease or damage is advancing.

CHAPTER 5

The All-American Diet Is a Liver Destroyer

O ur traditional all-American diet is, in many ways, a liver killer. Numerous studies have shown that this diet not only harms the liver; it is a major cause of heart attacks and strokes, the development of atherosclerosis (the disease process that causes heart and blood vessel disease), plays a major role in virtually all of the neurodegenerative diseases, and reaps havoc on the intestines and colon.

Known also as the Western diet, such foods include excessive red meat, processed and prepackaged foods, margarine, sweets (candy, pastries, cakes, and other desserts), both high-fat and low-fat dairy products, refined grains, potatoes, corn, pasta, breads, refined sugar, and, worst of all, fructose, especially high-fructose corn syrup.

These foods damage your liver because they fuel obesity, promote inflammation, induce insulin resistance and diabetes, contain excitotoxic additives, impair immunity, contain toxic additives, and are deficient in critical nutrients.

Traditionally, much of the research on the harmful impact of this traditional American diet has focused on parts of the body other than the liver, particularly the cardiovascular system and brain. Chronic inflammation induced by the Western diet has been strongly linked to coronary heart disease, type 2 diabetes, insulin resistance, metabolic syndrome, energy failure, and several neurodegenerative diseases, such as Alzheimer's disease and Parkinson's disease. The high content of gluten in the Western diet induces gluten sensitivity disorders. Processed food contains additives that promote cancer induction, organ degeneration, mitochondrial disruption, and a host of other cellular abnormalities. In addition, these foods frequently contain pesticide and herbicide residues that are not only toxic to the liver, but can also induce cancer. Carrageenan, a frequently used additive in many foods, especially pastries, breads, and ice cream, is a powerful inflammatory agent and is used to enhance cancer growth and cancer invasion in experimental cancer studies. It is also used in studies to induce inflammation in test animals.

These are the components of our traditional American diet that contribute to liver damage:

- Excessively fatty foods
- Starchy foods high on the glycemic index and of high glycemic load
- Sugars (especially fructose and sucrose)
- Food additives and dyes (MSG, hydrolyzed protein extract, etc.)
- Artificial sweeteners (aspartame, Splenda, stevia, etc.)
- Gluten
- Lectins
- Toxic metals (lead, mercury, aluminum, and cadmium)

Fats and Oils

Fats are an important component of a healthy diet, but the type of fat makes all the difference in the world. Saturated fats have gotten a bad name, but they are not the most harmful fat. Dr. Robert Atkins, creator of the Atkins Diet, demonstrated that a high-fat, low-carbohydrate diet not only reduced cholesterol levels, but also reduced the risk of insulin resistance, type 2 diabetes, and stimulated significant fat weight loss.

Fats are essential components for a number of functions, such as cell membrane function, immunity regulation, control of ion trafficking in cells, supporting inflammation mechanisms, controlling blood pressure, and for gene expression regulation (epigenetics). They are also essential for brain function and are the precursors for several hormones. In fact, fats can even act like pharmaceutical drugs if used in particularly high concentrations and configurations.

The chemistry of fats can be quite involved, but, basically, fats (lipids and oils) are divided into **saturated fats, polyunsaturated fats**, and **monounsaturated fats**. Each has a special function in the body. Polyunsaturated fats are divided into **omega-6 fats** and **omega-3 fats**. In limited amounts, the omega-6 fats are essential for good health. Yet, in excess they promote inflammation, cancer growth and the spread of cancer, neurodegeneration, and can severely damage organs and tissues, including the liver.

Omega-3 fats have a number of highly beneficial effects on health. They reduce inflammation, inhibit cancer growth and spread, are essential for brain function and protection, reduce atherosclerosis (heart attacks and strokes), reduce the impact and in some cases prevent autoimmune diseases, protect the intestines, are good for eyesight, and safeguard the heart. Recent studies have shown omega-3 oils to be very protective of the liver through a number of mechanisms.

Monosaturated oils are also generally healthy. Included in this classification is olive oil, which not only contains monounsaturated oil, but also special compounds from the olive that have several beneficial effects, such as anti-inflammatory effects, anticancer effects, and special effects that protect the liver. Olive oil contains high concentrations of fatty acid called *oleic acid* (*oleate*), which has powerful anticancer effects, especially against breast cancer. Oleate can also prevent palmitate, commonly found in saturated fats, from causing inflammation and insulin resistance. That is, mixing extra virgin olive oil and a saturated fat blocks the harmful effects of the saturated fat. Resveratrol (pterostilbene) also blocks palmitate toxicity.

Saturated fats generally contain fats in which all the double bonds that would make it susceptible to oxidation are removed (they are fully hydrogenated). In general, saturated fats, such as coconut oil, are much safer than any of the polyunsaturated omega-6 oils, such as corn, peanut, soybean, safflower, sunflower and canola oils.

Trans Fats

In 1910, the food industry introduced partially hydrogenated cooking oils to the market. Then, to make these oils more solid, they extended the process so that by 1911 they were able to manufacture a lard-like cooking fat called Crisco, which was partially hydrogenated as well. The problem with this process was that it generated a high percentage of **trans fats**, which were subsequently shown to have devastating health effects, including liver damage and the acceleration of atherosclerosis. It has been estimated that trans fats are responsible for 20,000 heart disease deaths annually. Since the 1970s, consumption of oils and fats in the U.S. increased by 62% with vegetable oils being the highest on the list.

Trans fats interfere with the ability of cell membranes to function—that is, they gum up the works. Several studies have shown that combining the food additive MSG with trans fats greatly increases the toxicity of the trans fats to the liver. This can lead to **steatohepatitis (NASH)** and eventually to primary liver cancer.

It took a great deal of effort by some determined researchers to finally get the government regulatory agencies interested in removing trans fats from food. Unfortunately, even labels that say "contains no trans fats" can be misleading, because many will still contain these harmful oils. If the label says "contains partially hydrogenated oils," it contains trans fats. Again, the only way to protect yourself is to prepare your own food fresh and avoid partially hydrogenated oils.

Polyunsaturated Oils

Most vegetable oils are omega-6 oils and are considered the type of oils most associated with inflammation, the stimulation of cancer growth, and tumor invasion in the liver. A high intake of these oils can significantly increase inflammation within the liver, resulting in nonalcoholic steatohepatitis (NASH), which can progress to liver fibrosis, liver cirrhosis, and a high incidence of hepatocarcinoma (primary liver cancer).

When omega-6 fats alone are fed to rats in high doses (as we see in humans consuming the Western diet), they develop a fatty liver, insulin resistance, diabetes, oxidative stress in the liver, inflammation, and elevated liver enzymes. In essence, these oils are a setup for serious liver disease in the future. One of the worst culprits containing omega-6 oils is margarine, which usually contains corn oil. Exposing the margarine to the air oxidizes the corn oil, and cooking with margarine is even worse, as heat greatly accelerates oxidation. Butter is preferable to margarine, as it will not oxidize.

The problem with polyunsaturated fats is that they are easily oxidized, and oxidized fats are extremely toxic, mainly by producing inflammation, free radicals, and lipid peroxidation products. This is a major problem with most processed foods, as they frequently contain omega-6 oils, such as peanut, corn, soybean, safflower, sunflower, and canola oils. Most salad dressings contain one or more of these oils and the most frequently used cooking oils include one of these oils. Many salad dressings will boldly say "contains olive oil" on the label, but in fine print adds that the dressing also contains the omega-6 oils. These oils should not be used in cooking and should be avoided in processed foods. The only way to avoid them is to prepare your own foods fresh.

Omega-3 oils, the other type of polyunsaturated oil, is also easily oxidized and should never be used as a cooking oil. Most omega-3 supplements are sealed to protect against oxidation. Omega-3 oils contain two types of components—one called **EPA** and the other **DHA**. Of the two components, the most useful in human health is the DHA, which can be purchased as a supplement. DHA within the body can be converted into several powerful anti-inflammatory compounds—**resolvins** and **protectins**.

Fats and Liver Diseases

While some researchers attributed eating a diet high in saturated fats as the cause of fatty liver diseases, more recent research has shown that saturated fats alone can cause a simple fatty liver, but it does not cause liver damage, fibrosis of the liver, or cirrhosis unless one's diet contains high levels of fructose or sucrose (table sugar). Sucrose is half glucose and half fructose. The strongest link to serious liver damage associated with fats is the high intake of fructose-sweetened sodas. In fact, studies have found that even in animals on a low-calorie diet, supplying high levels of fructose results in rapid onset of fatty liver disease (NAFLD). Fructose has been shown to stimulate fat formation within the liver, causes insulin resistance, triggers oxidative stress (high levels of free radicals and lipid peroxidation products), and induces liver inflammation. Fructose consumption has doubled over the past 30 years.

One Australian study of adolescents who consumed a typical Western diet, examined the children at age 14 and then again when they were 17 years old. A Western diet was considered to contain a high intake of soft drinks, refined grains, red meats, full fat dairy products, fast foods, processed meats, sauces, and dressings. The study found that 15.2% of the adolescents developed a fatty liver (nonalcoholic fatty liver disease—NAFLD). This increased to 52% by age 17 in boys who were overweight or obese. The foods most associated with NAFLD included soft drinks, sauces, and dressings. Most of the sauces and dressings contained polyunsaturated omega-6 oils and sugar (especially high-fructose corn syrup).

One of the strongest links to fatty liver damage associated with inflammation (NASH) is one's degree of **visceral fat**— that is, fat accumulating within the abdomen, surrounding your intestines, liver, and pancreas. This special fat triggers significant inflammation throughout the body and especially within the liver. A combination of MSG (a common food additive) and trans fatty acids (partially hydrogenated vegetable oils) has been shown to induce an especially severe inflammation, liver fibrosis, and insulin resistance (leading to type 2 diabetes).

When the liver is inflamed, it begins to malfunction, fat accumulation progresses, scar tissue begins to form (fibrosis), metabolism of one's food is disrupted, and eventually the liver damage becomes so severe (cirrhosis) that the liver begins to fail—death soon ensues. A scarred, cirrhotic liver is more likely to develop primary liver cancer (hepatocarcinoma).

Tips to Cut Down on Fat

- Make your own salad dressings using organic extra virgin olive oil.
- Use half-and-half instead of cream (or avoid milk altogether).
- Reduce your cheese intake.
- Substitute olive oil or coconut oil for cooking and add turmeric to the oil to prevent oxidation.
- Reduce your red meat intake; eat more low-mercury fish, poultry, and pork.
- Avoid processed food—make you own foods fresh and buy organically raised meats.
- Grill, bake, boil, steam, or casserole meals instead of frying.
- Avoid fatty desserts.
- Avoid pizza and many Mexican and Italian dishes that are high in fats.

Starchy Foods

Starches are complex carbohydrates such as potatoes, pasta, breads, rice, and grains. Sugars are considered simple carbohydrates and include glucose, fructose, galactose, and sucrose, for example. Starches eventually are broken down in the body into simple sugars or stored as glycogen, a complex of sugar molecules stored in the muscles and mainly in the liver. This food type is considered a source of quick energy, and various complexes of carbohydrates are used to construct complex molecules for cells and special tissue components.

Some starches are very quickly broken down into sugars and rapidly metabolized. We call these **high-glycemic** carbohydrates. Other starches are slowly broken down into sugars. We call these **low-glycemic** carbohydrates. The high glycemic carbohydrates trigger a rapid, and rather intense, insulin response, which can cause **reactive hypoglycemia**—a rapid fall in blood sugar. The low glycemic carbohydrates have a less intense insulin response and are slowly metabolized. High insulin levels promote fat deposition in tissues.

The most toxic of the sugars is fructose, but even glucose can have some toxicity to the liver and brain, especially if blood levels are elevated. Fructose, unlike the other sugars, causes no insulin response.

Central to the worst of the liver damage associated with a high-fat, high-fructose diet is the induction of inflammation within muscles, which is the main place glucose is metabolized. Muscle tissue is also the principal site of insulin's action, and inflammation can severely interfere with the ability of insulin to work—that is, it leads to **insulin resistance** and ultimately to **type 2 diabetes**. In fatty liver disease, large amounts of free fatty acids are released into the blood and ultimately find their way into the muscles, where they interfere with insulin's function. This can make a person a type 2 diabetic.

Starchy foods are our body's main source of carbohydrates, and it's a food group we need. The problem is that we usually eat too much of the "white" stuff, which is the highly processed type of foods such as white bread, rice, and pasta, which can raise blood sugar more than whole grains due to their lack of fiber. Fiber slows the absorption of sugars and carbohydrates. Fructose is strongly linked to developing the metabolic syndrome (called *syndrome X* in the past).

The metabolic syndrome is a cluster of conditions that include obesity, high cholesterol levels, abnormal blood lipids, and insulin resistance. All these conditions are thought to arise from a combination of inflammation and insulin resistance. Insulin resistance is linked to inflammation as well. What we begin to see is that there is a strong link between certain types of fats and fructose that results in inflammation and, eventually, all the conditions associated with abuse of these food components. Hypertension is commonly associated with the metabolic syndrome.

It is best to avoid all breads or at least severely limit the amount you have in your diet. While white bread is definitely bad, whole-grain breads, are in some ways much worse, because they are high in lectins, gluten, and glutamate (an excitotoxin). Those with gluten sensitivity should avoid all whole-grain breads.

Rice when purchased from the grocery store is not a good choice, because all rice is contaminated with arsenic—brown rice being the most contaminated. To remove the arsenic requires overnight soaking in purified water and repeated washings. Even purified, it is a high glycemic starch. There are now several alternatives to white rice such as quinoa, couscous, and farro. All of these substitutes contain some drawbacks and are best omitted from one's diet.

Sugar

Now, it's likely you know that sugar is bad for you—but you may not know how bad it is. Of course, the type of sugar matters in terms of toxicity. Glucose is far less toxic than fructose.

Here's the latest research:

- Sugar is now considered the major cause of obesity, which leads not only to diabetes and heart disease, but is also implicated in other chronic ailments, including several types of cancer. Fructose is far more fattening than other sugars (especially high-fructose corn syrup).

- Sugar fuels inflammation and insulin resistance, which is the driver in heart disease, strokes, atherosclerosis, and neurodegenerative diseases, as well as damage to other organs—your liver included! Again, fructose is more harmful for all these conditions than other sugars.
- Consuming too much sugar on a regular basis triggers eventual reactive hypoglycemia. This can lead to a number of health problems, including brain damage.
- Insulin resistance, as caused by fructose and sucrose, is linked to dementia. It is now suspected that in cases of Alzheimer's disease, we may be seeing a type of insulin resistance, which is now called "type 3 diabetes," similar to type 2 diabetes that we are familiar with, except it appears to be isolated within the brain. In fact, blood sugar outside the brain can be perfectly normal. We also know that high concentrations of glucose are toxic to brain cells (called *glucotoxicity*).
- Sugar is known to be highly addictive, so the more of it you eat, the more of it you crave.

Also, sugar is not only a major cause of obesity, but also metabolic syndrome, neurodegenerative diseases, reactive hypoglycemia, and contributes to all inflammatory diseases. And don't be fooled by the claim that it's only "refined" sugar that's the enemy, and that other forms, such as raw sugar, brown sugar, honey, and molasses, are okay. This is false. Sugar is sugar, and all sugar is a source of all these disorders. The best that can be said of these other forms of sugar, such as honey, maple syrup, and molasses, is that they also contain other compounds that promote our health.

What About Artificial Sweeteners?

Unfortunately, if you are addicted to artificial sweeteners—especially in sodas—you aren't doing your liver any good.

The reason people started using artificial sweeteners as a sugar replacement was to lose weight, but over the past few years, mounting research reveals this idea is a fallacy—especially when it comes to diet sodas, because research finds that people who drink diet soda have both larger waistlines and a higher risk of diabetes, metabolic syndrome, and NAFLD.

The exception may be stevia, which is a naturally occurring sweetener extracted from the stevia plant. Some preliminary research has found that this substance may actually provide liver benefits. But stevia has its problems as well, including toxicity to reproductive cells and to the brain.

One of the better and healthier nonnutritive sweeteners is monk fruit extract. One of its chief advantages being that it reduces inflammation.

It's obvious that the sweet taste in candy, soda, and cake comes from sugar, but do you know the other foods in which sugar is hiding? It's estimated that 50% of the sugar consumed by Americans is hidden in prepackaged foods or in foodstuffs you'd never suspect. Even toothpaste can be sweetened with sugar!

Adding sweet foods and drinks to your diet stimulates receptors in your brain that can drive insulin release just like real sugar, just not as intensely. Sweeteners can have profound effects on addiction centers in the brain, which make it difficult to trim the intake of real sugar and high glycemic carbohydrates.

Ways to Cut Down on Sugar

- **Cut out the obvious offenders.** Banish the sugar bowl, soft drinks, candy, etc., from your house, car, and office!

- **Be a label reader.** There are some 50 names that sugar can hide under. Here are some of the most common. Watch for these in various products' "ingredients" sections: lactose, brown rice syrup, molasses, dextrose, cane sugar, corn sweetener, corn sweetener solids, fructose, glucose, maltose, rice syrup, cane juice crystals, evaporated cane juice, raw sugar, organic raw sugar, maltodextrin, and many others.
- **Don't buy any foods that contain high-fructose corn syrup (HFCS).** This common sweetener in sodas and fruit-flavored drinks is manufactured in a way that turns its glucose into fructose, a type of sugar that is actually sweeter.
- **Make sure you're actually hungry, not thirsty.** Sugar cravings can be a sign you're dehydrated.
- **Get enough sleep.** Research finds that people who are tired tend to crave junk foods including sugar. Depression also enhances the craving for sugar.
- **Banish alcohol.** The problem with sugar is that it's addictive—so is alcohol. Not only are cocktails packed with sugar, but also alcohol can weaken your resolve to lay off other sweet items.
- **If your sweet tooth absolutely craves a fix, eat a few small squares of dark chocolate.** The higher the percentage of dark chocolate in the product, the lower the sugar content, as opposed to milk chocolate, which contains added sugar and fat.

Salt

Your body needs some salt. Known also as sodium chloride, salt helps maintain your body's balance of fluid.

The problem is that the government recommendation for salt intake is less than 2,300 milligrams a day, and while that sounds like a lot, it's basically about a teaspoon of salt, and most people get far more than that.

The natural salt in food accounts for about 10% of total intake, on average, according to the guidelines. The salt we add at the table or while cooking adds another 5 to 10%. About 75% of our total salt intake comes from salt added to processed foods by manufacturers, and salt that cooks add to foods at restaurants and other food-service establishments.

For some people, salt contributes to high blood pressure. High blood pressure makes the heart work harder and can lead to heart disease, stroke, heart failure, and kidney disease. Salt-sensitive hypertension makes up only a small percentage of cases of high blood pressure. Extreme salt restriction is dangerous and unnecessary. Excess salt can worsen neurological diseases based on its effects on neuron physiology.

Salt can also directly affect the liver in two ways. First, high blood pressure is one of the diseases that makes up the constellation of conditions in metabolic syndrome, and second, some research shows that too much sodium can lead to liver scarring, a precursor to cirrhosis.

Here are tips for cutting your salt intake:

- **Use your saltshaker sparingly.**
- **Eat whole, fresh foods.** Choose organic foods whenever possible. Packaged and processed foods are often packed with salt, not only for flavor but also as a preservative.
- **Learn to flavor foods with lemon juice, black pepper, ginger, fennel, bay leaves, rosemary, ginger, and garlic, instead of salt.** Be careful with salt substitutes—some are a blend that includes salt (called "sodium" on labels) or they may contain potassium chloride, which is not safe for people

with kidney problems. So, you may want to check with your doctor first.

- **Don't assume that sweets are salt-free.** Products meant to taste sweet, such as candy, cake mixes, and instant puddings, may all contain salt. Salt is added to a great number of processed foods.

- **Banish condiments.** Salt is often hiding in condiments, such as ketchup, barbecue sauce, meat tenderizers, and—especially—soy sauce.

- **Snack smartly.** Chips, pretzels, and crackers get their taste (and addictive quality) from salt. Substitute fresh veggies, or, for a treat, unsalted or lower-sodium versions of your favorites.

- **Pick fresh veggies (or frozen).** Fresh vegetables are your best choice. When not available, choose frozen. Canned vegetables are often prepared with salt, and sometimes sugar as well.

- **Beware fat-free or sugar-free foods.** When ingredients like fat and sugar are eliminated, manufacturers usually add salt to compensate.

- **Avoid extreme low-salt diets** because they can lead to severe salt depletion, which can cause severe illness and it is extremely difficult to restore needed salt content safely. Such diets are frequently used to treat poorly controlled hypertension. There are far safer natural ways to control elevated blood pressure, such as hawthorn, Nano-Grape Seed extract, high-dose vitamin C, magnesium, and Bonito fish extract.

CHAPTER 6

Is Your Lifestyle Putting Your Liver at Risk?

As you've seen, your liver is a repository for detoxifying and removing harmful substances, both from our environment and that generated by our own bodies. Normally, we think of these as pollution, such as pesticides, herbicides, fungicides, pharmaceutical drugs, toxic metals, and harmful food additives. But in many cases, they consist of harmful substances that we expose ourselves to, such as tobacco smoke, alcohol, toxic metals from canned goods, contaminated drinking water, chemicals from plastics, and other "miracles" of modern chemistry. It is human nature to ignore things we cannot see or taste, but these contain a number of toxic substances.

Normally, we think of these harmful substances entering us by eating or drinking, which does account for a great deal of the problem. Yet, you also have to include things that are inhaled, absorbed through the skin, and medications injected by medical personnel. Unfortunately, we must also include illicit drugs, which are now widely used by virtually all age groups.

By changing your lifestyle to one that is healthy, you also are protecting yourself from a number of diseases, such as heart disease, several types of cancer, and many other chronic diseases as well, including diabetes, stroke, kidney disease, high blood pressure, chronic lung disease, gastrointestinal diseases, neurodegenerative diseases, and many other deadly and life-altering diseases.

It is also important to keep in mind that all cells also contain detoxification systems, even though the liver is the body's main detoxification system. In general, when you strengthen your liver detoxification, you strengthen your cellular detoxification as well.

Smoking

Lighting a cigarette creates over 4,000 harmful chemicals, which have hazardous adverse effects on almost every organ in your body.

While most of us think of the damage by smoking affecting mostly the throat and the lungs, it also leads to systemic damage throughout the body, affecting many organs, including the liver. Tobacco smoke damages the arteries and causes them to narrow by drastically accelerating atherosclerosis. Keep in mind that smoking tobacco is highly inflammatory and generates massive amounts of free radicals throughout the body, even the brain. Smoking is a potentially lethal, and highly addictive disorder. Lifetime smokers have a 50% probability of dying due to tobacco-related causes, and, on average, will reduce their life expectancy by 10 years.

Smokers are at greater risk of a wide variety of chronic diseases beyond the respiratory system. In addition, smoking impacts the liver in many ways.

Research links cigarette smoking to accelerated disease progression in patients with chronic hepatitis C and B and those with other inflammatory liver diseases, such as cirrhosis. Smoking also appears to worsen liver injury in alcoholic liver disease and fatty liver disease, both nonalcoholic fatty liver disease (NAFLD), and in nonalcoholic steatohepatitis (NASH), which is a far more aggressive and potentially deadly form of fatty liver disease. Anything that promotes inflammation and free radical generation in the liver will worsen other liver diseases. This includes smoking.

Researchers have also looked at the impact of smoking on the alcoholic liver and found that excessive alcohol consumption can be particularly dangerous when combined with smoking. Indeed, the two habits often go together. These researchers found that, although smoking did not directly affect the function of the liver, it did enhance the detrimental effects of alcohol.

Smoking also increases the risk of liver cancer. Former smokers have a lower risk than current smokers, but both groups have a higher risk than those who have never smoked. Again, this makes sense because most cancers are caused by chronic inflammation. Hepatitis viruses, NASH, liver fibrosis, and cirrhosis are all associated with significant liver inflammation. Smoking magnifies this inflammation.

Smoking damages the liver by another mechanism that is often overlooked. Extensive research demonstrates that nicotine in tobacco smoke is a powerful inhibitor of the immune system, which greatly increases the risk of acquiring a liver infection, such as viral hepatitis, as well as bacterial and fungal liver infections. In addition, chronic immune suppression greatly increases the risk of developing a cancer, not just in the liver, but anywhere in the body—including brain cancers. When the immune system is suppressed, cancers grow faster and spread wider. Along these lines, it should be appreciated that statin cholesterol-lowering drugs are also powerful immune suppressors.

You may think that e-cigarettes are a healthier choice, but research is finding this is not true, both in terms of the impact on the body, and also directly on the liver. Vaping can cause severe damage to the lungs, leading to chronic hypoxia (low oxygen), and this can damage the liver as well. Research has also shown vaping smoke contains several toxic metals as well.

E-cigarette aerosol contains propylene glycol, which is metabolized in the liver into propionaldehyde, which is related to formaldehyde. When propionaldehyde accumulates in the body, it increases the potential for liver damage and is associated with the development of brain cancers.

Alcohol Use

We may enjoy drinking alcohol, but to our liver, it is, in reality, consuming a poison on a regular basis. Most alcohol, after being absorbed in the digestive tract, is processed (metabolized) in the liver. As alcohol is processed, substances that can damage the liver are produced. The more alcohol a person drinks, the greater the damage to the liver.

The overindulgence of liquor directly results in three types of liver damage, which can also be looked at as occurring in these three stages, starting as fat that accumulates in the liver and ending as cirrhosis.

These conditions that are directly linked to ingesting too much alcohol are:

- **Fat accumulation (hepatic steatosis).** Too much alcohol can result in fat forming in the liver. This occurs in more than 90% of people who drink too much alcohol, but it can usually be reversed when people quit drinking. Drinking a very large amount of alcohol rapidly (binge drinking) can result in a rapidly developing fatty liver, and in some cases can result in massive liver destruction and death within minutes, especially if one has preexisting liver damage.

- **Alcoholic hepatitis.** The word "hepatitis" means inflammation, and this is the type of hepatitis that is brought about by drinking. Alcoholic hepatitis is usually brought on by drinking too heavily over several years. The relationship between drinking and this disease is not that clear-cut—sometimes people who are heavy drinkers don't develop this condition, and sometimes it can occur in people who don't drink heavily. It's estimated that this condition occurs in about 10 to 35% of people who are chronic, heavy drinkers. One's nutritional status determines the degree of toxic damage by the alcohol, especially the intake of water-soluble vitamins, such as the B-complex vitamins, vitamin B_{12}, and folate. These vitamins offer considerable protection for the liver.

- **Cirrhosis.** About 10 to 20% of people who are chronic heavy drinkers will develop cirrhosis, a life-threatening condition in which healthy liver cells are replaced by scar tissue. Scar tissue cannot function in the place of liver cells. Eventually, the liver shrinks. Unlike fatty liver and alcoholic hepatitis, advanced cirrhosis cannot be reversed.

Any amount of alcohol can cause some damage to the liver. However, in an otherwise healthy person with no underlying liver problems, the probability of developing liver disease increases if a person drinks more than about 1.5 ounces of alcohol a day (especially if they drink more than about 3 ounces) for more than 10 years. Combining certain liver toxic substances, such as Tylenol (acetaminophen) or liver toxic prescription drugs, can make the liver much more sensitive to damage by alcohol. Anything that depletes the liver's glutathione, such as acetaminophen, lead, or mercury, will increase the liver's sensitivity to toxic substances. Glutathione levels, the body's main protective molecule, begins to decline progressively after age forty. This major cell protector is also depleted by chronic inflammation. Glutathione also significantly protects against viral infections.

One and one-half ounces of liquor a day is comparable to drinking about three cans of beer, three glasses of wine, or three shots of hard liquor. Men who develop cirrhosis typically drink more than about 3 ounces of alcohol a day for more than 10 years. Consuming 3 ounces a day involves drinking six cans of beer, five glasses of wine, or six shots of liquor. About half the men who drink more than 8 ounces of alcohol a day for 20 years develop cirrhosis.

Drinking on an empty stomach greatly increases the toxic effect of the alcohol. Wine, unlike hard liquor, contains beneficial substances from the grapes that protect the liver, such as resveratrol. The content of resveratrol in wine varies with the brand. Wine made from grapes grown on a mountaintop have much higher resveratrol levels than wine made from grapes grown in a valley. In addition, most wines contain high levels of sulfites and fluoride, both of which are significantly toxic, especially the fluoride. The fluoride content of wines also varies considerably. European wines generally have significantly lower fluoride levels than American wines.

Beer contains high levels of lectins, which can harm cells and worsen arthritis. It is also quite high in gluten from the barley and other grains used in brewing. Another danger from drinking beer, beyond the alcohol content, is that most are bottled in aluminum cans or aluminum kegs. Being acidic, beer can leech out the aluminum in large amounts. Usually, aluminum cans have special coatings to prevent leeching of aluminum, but these coatings are often broken or have gaps in them. The grains used in brewing are also high in glutamate, an excitotoxin.

Both men and women can experience liver damage from alcohol, but women are more vulnerable, even after adjusting for their smaller body size. It's been found that men are able to clear alcohol more efficiently than women. Women are at risk of liver damage if they drink about half as much alcohol as men. That is, drinking more than 0.75 to 1.5 ounces of alcohol a day puts women at risk. Risk may be increased in women because their digestive system may be less able to process alcohol, thus increasing the amount of alcohol reaching the liver, according to some research.

Beer and wine are not "safer" than whiskey or spirits if a person has an underlying liver condition such as hepatitis B or C, or prior damage from alcohol or other diseases. Under such conditions, the liver is very sensitive to any amount of alcohol. In those situations, the only safe course is abstinence.

Obesity

Excess weight has long been recognized as harmful to the body for many reasons, mainly because obesity is associated with high levels of inflammation in the body. Being overweight, and especially being obese, puts a person at very high risk of developing insulin resistance (type 2 diabetes), hypertension, depression, brain disorders, accelerating atherosclerosis, increased complications from infections, and the metabolic syndrome—all of which can shorten life. In recent years, however, it's also been discovered that excess weight can damage many internal organs.

Researchers have also discovered another explanation for how excess weight harms our internal organs, including possibly the liver. We used to think that excess fat was inert, but excess fat is also harmful on a molecular level. These researchers suggest that overeating may trigger the immune response, which causes chronic bodily inflammation, which, in turn, can damage the body. The worst fat is called **visceral fat**, which is fat accumulating within your abdomen, surrounding your intestines, colon, and other abdominal organs. While the so-called pot belly or beer belly is highly suspicious for having this inflammatory fat, people can have perfectly flat stomachs and still have excessive visceral fat. This fat causes intense inflammation within the liver, as well as the rest of the body. The damage is done through the release of high levels of inflammatory cytokines, chemokines, and other inflammatory chemicals from fat cells and infiltrating immune cells (mainly macrophages).

Obesity and being overweight is also the driving force behind nonalcoholic fatty liver disease (NAFLD) and nonalcoholic steatohepatitis (NASH), which is a more severe liver disorder that can destroy the liver and even trigger the development of a primary liver cancer (hepatocarcinoma). More about these two diseases in Chapter 13.

Sedentary Lifestyle

We are becoming a nation of coach potatoes, and our livers pay the price.

The federal government's physical activity guidelines for adults recommend that adults participate in some type of muscle strengthening activity at least twice a week, paired with moderate aerobic exercise for 150 minutes per week or 75 minutes per week of vigorously working out. Like most government recommendations, it is designed as if everyone were a widget stamped out of a common mold.

Exercise should be graded depending on one's age and level of physical fitness. Walking, especially up an incline, has been shown to produce most of the health benefits associated with more rigorous exercises. Vigorous exercise, such as aerobics, generates very high levels of free radicals and lipid peroxidation products during, and for several hours after, the exercise, which can do a great deal of harm. One must prepare for such intense exercise by taking an assortment of antioxidants, such as vitamin C, B-complex vitamins, vitamin E (mixed tocopherols and mixed tocotrienols), R-lipoic acid, curcumin, and other antioxidant flavonoids. The more intense the exercise, the more antioxidants one may need.

The consequence is that our bodies suffer, including our livers. In particular, research finds that inactivity is a culprit in the development of nonalcoholic fatty liver disease. After a literature review, University of Missouri researchers found that physical inactivity was the primary cause of chronic diseases such as diabetes, obesity, and fatty liver disease and that even people who set aside time for exercise regularly but are otherwise sedentary, may not be active enough to combat these diseases.

Exercise without a healthy diet defeats the goal of better overall health and longevity. Harmful foods can make exercise either of little benefit or even more harmful. For example, if your diet is filled with sugars (especially fructose), breads, desserts, pro-inflammatory fats, and abundant processed foods, your body will be in a state of high oxidative stress, which could worsen the oxidative stress produced by aerobic exercise. These foods will also fill your body with a number of toxic compounds, which can put a lot of stress on your liver.

Toxic Food Dyes

Many foods contain various colorful food dyes, several of which have proven to be toxic. It is important to appreciate that the FDA allows the manufacturers of these dyes to conduct their own safety tests. Past experience, as with aspartame, has shown that many of these tests are manipulated to show that the products are "safe" and to hide any major harmful effects. Independent testing, when actually done, frequently shows major dangers.

The three most frequently used dyes, Red 40, Yellow 5, and Yellow 6 (90% of all the dyes used), each demonstrated problems, and recommendations from independent sources suggest they should never be used. These dyes are used in baked goods, beverages, dessert powders, candies, cereals, and many pharmaceutical drugs. Children consume amounts far greater than listed as safe by the FDA. As an example of toxicity, FD&C Yellow 5 (tartrazine) was shown to contain several carcinogens and DNA damaging compounds. Things are even worse today, because many of these food dyes are now coming from China, which does not have food safety regulations as stringent as other countries. Human studies found that 26% of people had hypersensitivity reactions to foods containing this dye. FD&C Red 40, the most commonly used food dye, was found to cause DNA damage, induced specific types of tumors, and contained a number of carcinogenic contaminants. Authors of the review suggested it should never be used in foods or pharmaceutical drugs.

The food dye FD&C Green 3 was shown to increase the incidence of bladder tumors, as well as tumors of the livers in experimental animals. FD&C Blue 2 food dye was associated with a significant increase in breast cancers and brain gliomas, and FD&C Red 1 dye was associated with an increase in liver cancers. FD&C blue 1 dye was associated with abnormal development of a child's brain. Children consume these dyes in much higher concentrations than adults, and because of their small size these dyes are much more toxic for them.

In my view, no one should consume foods or pharmaceutical products containing these dyes. Many foods contain several of these dyes, and studies have shown synergistic toxicity.

Exposure to Pesticides, Herbicides, and Fungicides

A number of chemical agents used in controlling pests and reducing the growth of weeds have been found to have profound deleterious effects on human health, especially in newborns, small children, and adolescents. One group of pesticides, called *organophosphorus pesticides*, has been shown even in low doses (less than will affect a bug) to cause damage to developing babies, newborns, and even adolescents. These pesticides disrupt the development of these children's brains. Studies have shown that following treatment of a house with a pesticide, residues of the chemical can be found on all surfaces in the house, including children's toys.

Interestingly, and of great concern, researchers found increased aggressiveness among male offspring exposed to chlorpyrifos, a major organophosphate pesticide. It is the liver that is responsible for detoxifying these compounds. One group of researchers looked at the effects of organophosphate pesticides on the liver of experimental animals.

They found that all of these compounds, such as malathion, parathion, diazinon, and chlorpyrifos, cause damage to the liver, even in doses that were low. This included significant structural damage to the cells in the liver, increases in inflammation, and areas of cell death. Their detailed examination discovered that these pesticides raised liver enzymes, impaired the flow of bile and bile excretion, raised cholesterol levels, suppressed ATP production, reduced glutathione in the liver and damaged the DNA of liver cells. Of major concern was the finding of several benign and malignant liver tumors in rats exposed to the pesticides.

These pesticides are being sprayed in homes, gardens, and public areas in addition to tons of such chemicals being used in agriculture. Unfortunately, schools—from preschools to universities and colleges—are exposing their students and teachers to these toxic compounds on a daily basis.

Pesticide and herbicide exposure has been linked to Parkinson's disease, and the most vulnerable individuals are considered to be those with poor detoxification. Other neurodegenerative diseases are also linked to pesticide and herbicide exposure, such as ALS and Alzheimer's disease.

Recently, scientists discovered that 30% of the breakdown products of these chemicals in the environment are more toxic than the actual parent compound. The U.S. Geological Survey recently conducted an examination of 442 small streams in urban and agricultural areas in five regions in the U.S., and after examining 3700 water samples, discovered that all of them contained pesticides, many with several pesticides. Worse, they found high levels of the toxic breakdown products in these streams and in the groundwater.

Herbicides, especially those containing glyphosate, are being used in enormous amounts all over the U.S. It has become America's favorite weed-control product. This is one of the most toxic compounds in use. Studies have shown that it has contaminated virtually everything. It has been found in groundwater, lakes, streams, reservoirs, foods, beverages, baby foods, vaccines, soils, playgrounds, public buildings, homes, and offices everywhere. This herbicide compound, a major ingredient in Roundup, has been proven to be a cancer-causing compound.

Fortunately, a number of safe pesticides can be used in gardens that contain no toxic chemicals. Pyrethrin, however, while naturally found, is linked to several types of cancer, especially in children. In my newsletters, I always suggest that my readers not use a pesticide service for their homes. Natural methods should be used to control household insects.

I will discuss pesticides, herbicides, and fungicides further in the next chapter.

CHAPTER 7

Food Additives and Artificial Sweeteners

If you have ever looked at the labels on processed foods, drinks, or soups, you will see a long list of additives that resemble names seen only in a chemistry textbook, such things as allyl anthranilate and benzyl dimethyl carbinyl butyrate. Remember, most of these compounds are foreign to the human body and must be detoxified or metabolized, mostly by your liver. More importantly, a number of these complex chemicals have never been adequately tested for long-term safety, especially when used together. Many such compounds have synergistic toxicity, meaning their toxicity exceeds just adding them together. By using them together the toxicity is greatly magnified.

These potentially, and even proven, toxic compounds have inundated our planet in such a way that virtually all are in danger of some degree of injury. Most supermarkets are filled with processed foods and drinks. In fact, virtually all the main shelves in these stores are brimming with these manufactured products, and more are on the way. The latest innovations in foods include manufactured meats and "meat glue." The latter is a process where less expensive cuts of meats are literally glued together, using special enzymes and a mixture high in toxic excitotoxins.

There is a heavy price to pay for all this "modern innovation" in foods. Until recently, our lifespans were increasing significantly. Studies starting around 2015, however, found that this trend seemed to be ending, and even going in reverse. Before this, there had been no decline in our lifespan since 1993. In fact, the highest increase in types of diseases has been neurodegenerative diseases.

When I was in medical school in the 1960s, degenerative diseases, such as multiple sclerosis, ALS, Alzheimer's dementia, Parkinson's disease, and seizures were relatively rare or at least "uncommon." Yet, each of these terrible disorders is on the rise, and in some countries, such as the U.S. and Great Britain, the increase is substantial. Microwave radiation from cell phones, cell phone towers, and the mass use of Wi-Fi has added considerably to this trend. Once 5G takes over the world, Heaven help us.

Most chemical food additives, household products, vaccines, agricultural chemicals, and industrial chemicals are inadequately tested. Many are never tested, and virtually all undergo testing only by the company that manufactures the chemical or product in question. Agencies, such as the Environmental Protection Agency (EPA) and the Food and Drug Administration (FDA), never conduct their own tests; they merely accept the tests performed by the companies being investigated. Products, chemicals, and even supplements manufactured in China are never inspected or tested at all. Inspectors from the FDA are not allowed to enter these Chinese facilities. American inspectors are forced to take the word of the Chinese governmental officials that all is well. This makes the world a much more dangerous place than ever before.

There is general agreement that a drastic change in our diets over the decades, with heavy doses of junk foods and other foods with poor nutritional content, also contributes heavily to our problems. In fact, our exposure to the sea of chemicals added to foods enhances the harmful effects of a poor diet, and vice versa. Many of these chemical additives drastically enhance inflammation, free radical generation, and lipid peroxidation—the very same things that a poor diet does as well.

What is truly frightening is that these bad diets and exposure to a massive amount of food additives begins even before birth, because pregnant women are also consuming and being exposed to these toxic compounds all though their pregnancies— what they eat, their babies are also exposed to. After birth, the child begins, in far too many cases, a lifetime exposure to all these harmful influences.

Here are some of the major harmful things most of us are exposed to, many of which are hidden in our foods and medicines.

Excitotoxins

The liver plays a Herculean task in nourishing and protecting the body, but today's modern life damages it in many ways through chemical exposures foreign to the body. One of the often-ignored ways we are destroying our own health is by consuming enormous amounts of these excitotoxic food additives. Most processed foods contain one or more excitotoxin additives.

Over the past 30 years I have been studying and writing about a toxic process called **excitotoxicity**. In 1995, I wrote a book about my findings called *Excitotoxicity: The Taste That Kills*.

Our brain contains a group of glutamate receptors that regulate the excitation of neurons in our nervous system. While glutamate is the most abundant neurotransmitter in the brain, ironically it is also the most toxic to the brain. It is for this reason that the brain possesses a multitude of mechanisms to keep the concentration of glutamate outside of cells at very low concentrations. It is the glutamate outside the cells that causes the problem.

Elevation of these glutamate levels outside of cells plays a major role in almost all neurodegenerative diseases (Alzheimer's dementia, Parkinson's disease, ALS, Huntington's disease, and many more), brain destruction from brain injuries, stroke damage, damage from meningitis, seizures, and damage from autoimmune diseases such as multiple sclerosis.

Excitotoxin food additives and foods naturally high in excitotoxins can, when eaten regularly, enter the brain and add to the damage done by these diseases. Exposure to these food additive excitotoxins early in life can cause the brain to develop abnormally and can result in neurological and other disorders later in life.

One recent startling discovery was that glutamate receptors exist on virtually all cells—bone cells, lung cells, kidneys, heart, muscles, gastrointestinal system cells, insulin producing cells in the pancreas, immune cells, and liver cells. What this means is that consuming food high in excitotoxic additives (such as MSG and aspartame) can damage every organ and tissue in the body, and not just the brain and spinal cord. We also know that excitotoxins dramatically increase inflammation, free radical generation, and lipid peroxidation—the main processes causing most diseases.

Excitotoxins and Liver Disorders

The liver's primary cell, the hepatocyte, contains a full assortment of glutamate receptors, just like brain cells, and overactivation of these receptors can trigger inflammation, scarring (fibrosis), and eventual destruction of these critical liver cells. Several studies have shown that excessive glutamate in the diet of animals can indeed trigger liver inflammation and liver cell destruction.

It has also been shown that exposing a pregnant animal to MSG can alter how the developing infant metabolizes fats in the liver, and that later in life—after reaching adulthood—the animal will have elevated cholesterol levels, as well as other fats associated with disease. In addition, they develop the same accumulation of fat in their livers that we see in NAFLD.

As you have seen earlier, one of the strongest connections to fatty liver disease and eventual cirrhosis is consumption of excessive amounts of fructose (especially high-fructose corn syrup). A recent study, by Dr. Kate Collison and coworkers, demonstrated that combining MSG with high-fructose consumption not only damaged the liver and caused a fatty liver, but also was one of the principal ways people accumulate visceral fat—the type of fat linked to numerous health problems, including the more devastating forms of fatty liver disease.

The excitotoxin–fructose combination doubled the amount of visceral fat and raised triglyceride and total cholesterol levels substantially. Triglycerides are more strongly associated with heart attacks and stroke risk than is cholesterol.

Most studies have shown that MSG can cause prolonged inflammation of the liver, even from a single dose. This increases the risk of developing cirrhosis and especially hepatocarcinoma (primary liver cancer). Keep in mind that the MSG absorbed from your diet travels directly to your liver by way of the hepatic portal blood supply, meaning it gets a very high concentration of the toxic glutamate.

In the Collison study, they found that the MSG alone could cause swelling of both the liver and the kidneys. The liver enzymes (ALT and AST) were significantly elevated by the MSG and serum albumin, and total proteins were significantly decreased, indicating significant liver damage by the MSG. Examination of the kidneys demonstrated significant damage by the MSG, leading to abnormal kidney function. Importantly, the MSG, as we saw earlier with fructose, also induced insulin resistance—which is the major link to type 2 diabetes.

Most people have been ingesting high levels of both fructose and glutamate food additives every day for decades. This keeps the liver in a state of constant inflammation and has it literally swimming in free radicals and lipid peroxidation products. These findings also explain why we are seeing a tremendous rise in the incidence of fatty liver disorders even in very small children.

The combination of high-fructose corn syrup (or high-sucrose intake) plus a high dietary glutamate intake dramatically worsens these liver destroying processes and can cause a simple fatty liver to progress to liver fibrosis (scarring) and finally cirrhosis of the liver, which leads to a need for a liver transplant. This combination also greatly increases one's risk of developing primary liver cancer (hepatocarcinoma), a highly fatal form of cancer.

As you will see later, a diet high in excitotoxin additives and fructose also significantly worsens the damage done by hepatitis viruses, such as the hepatitis C and hepatitis B viruses. The high level of inflammation caused by the combination, or even if either is used alone, will stimulate the growth and invasion of liver cancer—acting as a sort of cancer fertilizer.

It is important to appreciate that the dose of MSG used in the studies by Dr. Collison were 30 to 40 times lower than used in most MSG toxicity studies, meaning we are talking about glutamate levels commonly ingested by people eating diets high in processed foods. The amount of excitotoxin additives being added to foods have doubled every decade since they were first introduced.

Most of the damage produced within the liver by MSG and other glutamate food additives is caused by high levels of induced free radical and lipid peroxidation products, which explains why powerful antioxidants can significantly reduce this damage. There is an interaction between infiltrating immune cells and glutamate receptors within the liver, which magnifies the damage. I coined the name **immunoexcitotoxicity** to describe this devastating process. Basically, what is occurring is that as the damage from the glutamate begins, the immune system is activated, sending immune cells into the liver. These immune cells release special inflammatory factors (cytokines) that magnify the activation of glutamate receptors caused by the ingested glutamate or aspartate (aspartame) food additives. Together, these two processes do a great deal of damage to liver cells.

Studies have shown that powerful antioxidants, such as vitamin C and E, Nano-Curcumin, Nano-Quercetin, Nano-Silymarin, L-carnitine, as well as the B-complex vitamins, can all protect the liver against much of this damage—but not all of it. This means that you must stop eating foods with excitotoxin additives and avoid artificial sweeteners, such as aspartame and saccharin.

Hiding Excitotoxin Additives in Processed Foods

One of the first described adverse reactions to monosodium glu-tamate (MSG) was a condition called the Chinese restaurant syndrome. It was observed that certain people, when eating foods containing high levels of MSG, complained of severe headaches, tight neck muscles, a tight constriction in the center of the chest, diarrhea, and flushing of the face.

Dr. John Olney, a friend of mine, later discovered the brain damaging effects of MSG consumption. I visited his laboratory many years ago, when he was doing his primary studies. He showed me photomicrographs demonstrating the ability of MSG to destroy neurons in specific areas of the brain and the retina of the eye.

It was his testimony before a congressional committee on food safety that ended the practice by food processors of adding MSG to infant foods. Dr. Olney demonstrated that infants were many times more sensitive to the brain damaging effects of glutamate.

As news began to spread of the side effects of MSG, consumers insisted it be removed from foods. Food processors were reluctant to remove the MSG because it was a significant way to enhance the taste of foods. The maker of MSG and similar high-glutamate additives had a powerful vested interest in continuing the practice of adding these powerful compounds to foods, because this was a multibillion-dollar industry (located in Japan).

As a result of these two vested interests, food processors began to disguise the names of glutamate food additives and use food additives that were very high in glutamate levels besides MSG. Unfortunately, regulatory agencies allowed the food processors to engage in this deception and to even put on labels such as "Contains no MSG," when in fact they included high glutamate–containing additives that cause the very same damage. It is the glutamate in MSG and not the "monosodium" that causes the toxicity.

You should get in the habit of reading food labels and recognizing the primary hidden and disguised names for these excitotoxic food additives. It is a general principle that liquid forms of glutamate-containing foods do the greatest amount of damage—such as soups, soft drinks, sauces, and broth. This is because the glutamate in these foods is rapidly absorbed and reaches very high blood levels rapidly. The only sure way to avoid glutamate food additives is to avoid all processed foods and eat only foods you prepare fresh using organic foods.

A newer source of glutamate excitotoxins is in what have been called "meat glues." Meat glues utilize a special enzyme (transglutaminase) that is used to glue together cheaper cuts of meat that can resemble more expensive cuts. By adding a number of high glutamate–containing additives to the meat glue, food processors can make the manufactured food taste just like a higher price cut of meat. It is also used for cheeses, baked goods, and other foods. These meat glues, in my opinion, are just as harmful as MSG, and maybe more so.

Here are some of the more commonly used disguised names for high-glutamate food additives:

- Monosodium glutamate
- Hydrolyzed vegetable protein
- Hydrolyzed protein
- Hydrolyzed plant protein
- Plant protein extract
- Sodium caseinate
- Calcium caseinate
- Yeast extract
- Textured protein
- Autolyzed yeast
- Hydrolyzed oat flour
- Soy protein concentrate
- Soy protein isolate whey
- Protein concentrate
- Carrageenan enzymes (Protease enzymes from various sources can release excitotoxin amino acids from food proteins.)

The following additives almost always contain MSG:

- Malt extract
- Malt flavoring
- Bouillon broth
- Stock flavoring
- Natural flavoring

- Natural beef- or chicken-flavored seasoning spices
- Seasoning spices

Trans Fats, MSG, and Fatty Liver Disease

Dr. Collison and her coworkers performed a second study that brought considerably more light to the subject of fatty liver diseases. In this innovative study, they looked at the effect of combining a diet high in trans fats with MSG. Previously, it had been shown that excess dietary trans fats could cause obesity and insulin resistance—both are linked to a fatty liver. It was also estimated that diets high in trans fats were responsible for 20,000 excess cardiovascular deaths in the U.S. alone, and that insulin resistance and obesity were strongly linked to cardiovascular deaths as well. As in their previous study, they used doses of MSG that were well within what most people were consuming in their diets.

It has been shown that both MSG and trans fats could cause a significant increase in visceral fat—the deadliest form of fat. In their study, they fed rats either a low dose of MSG or a diet high in trans fats. A third group was fed a combination of MSG plus the trans fat diet. Control mice ate the standard low-fat chow.

They found that the rats eating the MSG additive diet developed a significant increase in visceral fat, as did the animals eating the diet containing the trans fat. But when MSG was combined with the trans fat diet, the animals developed massive amounts of visceral fat. This finding is very important, because increased amounts of visceral fat are a predictor of risk for developing steatohepatitis (NASH), the form of fatty liver that is most associated with eventual liver failure and primary liver cancer. They also found that the combination resulted in very high levels of free fatty acids and triglycerides in the blood, things that are linked to a very high risk of cardiovascular diseases, such as heart attacks and strokes.

As with most things done by regulatory agencies, in the case of trans fats one cannot trust the assurances of "low" or "no trans fats" appearing on food labels. As I mentioned before, food labels can say that the product contains "no trans-fats" but still contain considerable trans fats. If a food contains **partially hydrogenated vegetable oil**, it contains significant amounts of trans fats.

Aspartame

Aspartame is one of the most commonly used artificial sweeteners in the world. Chemically, it is a methyl-ester of two common amino acids: L-phenylalanine and L-aspartic acid (an excitotoxin). When metabolized, aspartame is broken down into its two main amino acids and the highly toxic alcohol, methanol. Methanol is further metabolized to produce the extremely toxic chemical formaldehyde (commonly known as an *embalming fluid*).

Formaldehyde binds very tightly to proteins in the tissues, severely disrupting their function (called *protein adducts*) and causing DNA damage. Because formaldehyde binds so tightly to proteins, it tends to accumulate each time aspartame is consumed. Over time, considerable damage is done to organs and tissues. In addition, formaldehyde is a powerful carcinogen, strongly linked to brain cancers.

In the real world, people commonly consume both aspartame and MSG (or other excitotoxic food additives) together. One study looked specifically at what happens when these two substances are added together. What they found was that when MSG and aspartame were combined in doses used in real-world situations, they significantly increased fat in the liver (triglycerides) and caused the highest increase in visceral fat among all other diet combinations. Keep in mind that high visceral fat levels also increase the incidence of such diseases as sleep apnea, cardiovascular disease (heart attacks and strokes), liver failure, and even degenerative brain diseases.

Combining MSG, aspartame, and trans fats creates a nightmare situation that is almost beyond imagination. The effect of trans fats is so powerful that it has been shown that visceral fat is increased substantially even when experimental animals were on an otherwise low-fat or low-calorie diet. It has been shown that combining aspartame, MSG, and trans fats together raised blood sugar the highest, and as expected, insulin resistance was also significantly increased. This would certainly explain the high incidence of type 2 diabetes among Americans who regularly follow such a diet combination. In addition, consuming both MSG and aspartame significantly increased inflammation.

It has also been shown that MSG makes it much easier to induce diabetes in animals when they are obese, and adding aspartame adds considerably to this devastating combination.

Several studies have been done to evaluate the effect of chronic aspartame consumption on the liver. One such study found that chronic use of aspartame caused significant damage to liver cells and to the kidney as well. In this study, researchers found very high levels of **lipid peroxidation** in the liver—that is, oxidation of the lipids in liver cells—a very harmful effect. They also found higher levels of **nitric oxide** and very low **glutathione** levels in the liver. Keep in mind that glutathione is one of the most important chemicals used to protect all cells, especially liver cells. Low levels of glutathione puts the liver at great risk for severe damage by any toxic substance. Glutathione neutralizes the superoxide free radicals, nitric oxide, hydroxyl radicals, and peroxynitrite, making it one of our most important cell protectors. If all this was not bad enough, the researchers also found high levels of DNA fragmentation, which increases the risk of developing liver cancer.

We hear a lot about the beneficial effects of nitric oxide, but this compound is a double-edged sword. It has some very beneficial functions, but under certain conditions it is also involved in severe inflammation and excitotoxicity. Nitric oxide becomes very harmful under conditions of high free radical formation, because it rapidly combines with the free radical superoxide to form the extremely harmful radical called *peroxynitrite*. This is what happens with excitotoxicity and during inflammation.

Another study found that a daily intake of aspartame for 2 to 6 weeks in animals causes a dramatic increase in liver lipid peroxidation and a drastic fall in a number of critical antioxidant enzymes, such as superoxide dismutase (SOD), catalase (CAT), and glutathione (GSH). This leaves the liver vulnerable to all toxic substances a person may be exposed to, making the risk of developing advanced liver disease or even liver cancer much higher. Keep in mind that all of us are constantly exposed to tens of thousands of toxic compounds from the environment, our food, and from medications. Aspartame and excitotoxic food additives, such as MSG, put us at a much higher risk than if we maintained a healthy liver. Their study also found similar damage to the kidneys due to aspartame.

It appears from all these studies that the most harmful compound in aspartame is methanol. Methanol levels rise very rapidly after a single ingestion of aspartame. And, gradually, the methanol is metabolized into an even more harmful compound: formaldehyde.

Aspartame has also been shown to be harmful to developing babies should the mother consume aspartame while pregnant.

More studies are appearing demonstrating the harmful effects of aspartame on other organs, such as the brain, the immune system, the kidneys, and the heart. For example, studies have shown that long-term consumption triggers high levels of damaging lipid peroxidation within the brain. Because the brain is composed of a very high level of lipids, this puts the brain at very high risk and probably explains the high incidence of brain tumors associated with aspartame in animal studies.

The effect of aspartame on the heart is truly frightening. In one study, researchers found a significant elevation of lipid peroxidation within the heart muscle and a significant decline in all the heart's antioxidant enzymes, including glutathione. This represents the worst situation one can imagine—high levels of free radical generation, but a severe deficiency in antioxidant defenses. Examination of the heart muscle demonstrated areas of dead tissue and microscopic hemorrhages, along with considerable DNA damage within heart cells. The harmful effects on the heart were dose dependent, meaning the higher the intake of aspartame, the worse the damage. Worse still is the knowledge that the damage is accumulative, meaning the longer one drinks aspartame sodas, the greater the damage. Even one aspartame sweetened soda a day can do significant damage.

Aspartame has been shown to cause high levels of inflammation and free radical, lipid peroxidation damage in all lymphoid organs—lymph nodes, spleen, and thymus gland. It also causes damage to white blood cells, all of which explains the high incidence of lymphomas in experimental animals exposed to aspartame, as well as the same incidence in humans consuming this sweetener. One study demonstrated a dramatic fall in critical antioxidant enzymes within white blood cells, with the most devastating effect pertaining to lymphocytes—the most critical cell type in fighting viruses and cancer. This research also demonstrated that aspartame dramatically lowers vitamin C levels in immune cells, which puts one at a very high risk of free radical injury.

Approximately 70% of all aspartame consumed comes from sodas. It is also used to sweeten many medications, especially those designed for children. In my opinion, it should have been banned when it was first proposed. Considerable evidence demonstrated that the FDA was influenced to approve this dangerous sweetener despite clear evidence it was far too dangerous to be used as a sweetener. This mistake needs to be corrected.

Saccharin as Compared to Aspartame

There is no question aspartame is a very harmful substance linked to many types of damage, including several types of cancer. One study compared the toxicity of aspartame to that of saccharin, and found saccharin to be even more harmful and damaging. The researchers used doses of aspartame and saccharin that conformed to expected human consumption.

Both sweeteners caused damage to the liver, raised liver enzymes, and caused considerable histological damage to the liver. In fact, microscopic examination showed areas of complete degeneration and the infiltration of immune cells, as well as obstruction of the microscopic veins the liver uses for transport. Saccharin produced greater DNA damage than did aspartame at comparable doses.

Protection Against Aspartame Toxicity

Aspartame has been shown to cause considerable damage to a number of organs, including the liver, kidneys, the heart, reproductive organs, and the brain. Fortunately, there are a number of natural compounds that can dramatically reduce the damage by aspartame. This should not be a call for one to continue this product because these protection studies are not complete.

One natural product, L-carnitine, has been shown to provide significant protection against damage both to the heart and the liver. Studies indicate that L-carnitine can reverse the severe suppression of glutathione by aspartame and also improve the level of other antioxidant enzymes as well, which reduces significantly all the factors causing the aspartame-induced damage. L-carnitine also significantly reduced the DNA damage caused by aspartame.

Selenium has been shown to protect the kidneys from damage by aspartame. However, a dose of selenium should be limited to 100 mcg a day.

All natural products that suppress oxidative stress, such as R-lipoic acid, Nano-Curcumin, Nano-Quercetin, Nano-Silymarin, Nano-Grape Seed extract and N-acetyl-L-cysteine (NAC), vitamin C, vitamin E, DHA, and magnesium will offer significant protection against liver damage by these chemicals.

CHAPTER 8

Liver Toxic Chemicals to Avoid

Most people feel comforted thinking that one or more of the federal or local regulatory agencies will protect them from harmful compounds and devices. Nothing could be further from the truth. A recent review of the regulatory process has shown that only 1% of the food supply is even examined for harmful substances.

Every minute of every day, we are exposed to tens of thousands of such industrial chemicals, as well as additives to our drinking water, microwave radiation exposure, and other harmful influences.

It is important to keep in mind that all these harmful influences are not only additive, but in many cases are synergistic. That is, rather than just adding the harmful effects together as you would for 2 + 2 equals 4, synergistic toxicity would have a multiplier effect on toxicity, as one would imagine 2 + 2 now equals 50.

This means that if you are exposed to a very low dose of a pesticide (a subtoxic dose) and a very low dose of a potentially toxic cleaning product, the result would be, within you, as if you were exposed to a full toxic dose.

We see this commonly in an exposure to two weak carcino-gens (cancer-causing chemicals), which alone will not cause can-cer but when combined in the same product will have the effect of being exposed to a powerful carcinogen. We also see this syn-ergistic toxicity with pesticides, herbicides, and fungicides, which are always used together. Even things not remotely related can have additive or synergistic toxicity if you are exposed to them at the same time.

One of the biggest flaws in safety testing is the fact that there is no agency testing for the effects of combining these toxic sub-stances. The public remains the largest group of experimental test subjects of all, but few regulators are actually studying the effects of combining these toxic compounds. Most toxicity studies are short-term studies. Few studies are done to look for the effects of long-term exposure. There are numerous instances of delayed effects occurring months, years, or even decades after the expo-sure to such compounds.

We also have to be concerned with bioaccumulation. A toxic compound that is not quickly detoxified or removed from the body will linger for months, years, or even a lifetime. What this means is that if we are exposed to the toxin on a regular basis, each dose accumulates so that a higher and higher dose devel-ops—eventually reaching a level that is maximally toxic.

Often, we are told that we can protect ourselves from these chemicals simply by washing contaminated vegetables with a veggie wash. Unfortunately, some of these agrichemicals are sys-temic pesticides, which are disseminated throughout the vegeta-ble—meaning they cannot be washed off. Some vegetables, such as bell peppers, cucumbers, avocados, and apples are coated with a wax to prevent spoilage. Often, pesticides are combined with this water-proof wax, which also cannot be washed off.

The highest concentration of pesticides is found on and in vegetables and some meats and include tomatoes, beef, potatoes, celery, kale, lettuce, oranges, apples, peaches, pork, wheat, soybeans, carrots, chicken, corn, and grapes.

There are over 65,000 chemicals in the Environmental Protection Agency's registry, the vast majority of which have not been adequately tested for toxicity, especially on the nervous system. Virtually none have been tested looking for effects on higher brain functions, such as learning, memory, cognitive processing, and the ability to think clearly and logically.

It has been estimated that more than nine million people have come into regular contact with known neurotoxins in the workplace, and tens of millions live with many of these chemicals in their homes. More than a thousand new chemicals are added every year to the existing stock of chemicals already used; most have been poorly tested. Added to this enormous figure, there are some two million chemical mixtures, blends, and other formulations already in use by industry. Over 60,000 of these chemicals are known to cause at least some neurological damage.

An incredible 1.2 billion pounds of pesticides are being used every year in the U.S., with over 600 types of pesticides in current use, 64 of these have been identified by the EPA as having carcinogenic potential. Worldwide, some four billion pounds of pesticides are used annually. These pesticides have been shown to enter the upper regions of our atmosphere and are spread all around the world, even to the remotest of areas. Pesticide residues have even been found in animals living in the Antarctic. In the U.S., these pesticides are being spread over 900,000 farms, equal to millions of acres.

It is telling that many cancers, especially lymphomas and leukemias, have their highest incidence among those living on farms. The same is true of several neurological disorders, such as Parkinson's and Alzheimer's disease.

If you think you are safe because you don't live on a farm, think again. We have a national obsession with having bug-free homes, and a large percentage of people use pesticide services to keep their houses bug-free or they use their own favorite bug spray. Perfect, weed-free lawns, are an equal obsession. Most of these outdoor herbicides are used during hot summer days. In the heat, these chemicals evaporate and can be drawn into homes by the ventilation system, combining the indoor pesticides with the outdoor herbicides—greatly magnifying the toxic effects.

Several studies have shown that children, even pets, who play in such yards have a significantly higher incidence of leukemia than normal. It is estimated that 150,000 to 500,000 pesticide-related illnesses are reported each year, with 200 people dying every year. Many more are crippled for life.

Numerous studies have shown that most important in preventing, or at least reducing, the harmful effects of these chemicals is the strength and health of our detoxification systems—that includes mainly our liver, but also the many detoxification systems within each of our cells as well. Of concern is that many of these chemicals can damage these critical detoxification systems themselves.

Anything that damages the liver itself—for example, aspartame, excitotoxin food additives, food dyes, fluoride (and fluoro-aluminum complexes), toxic metals, drugs, industrial chemicals, many agrichemicals, and chronic diseases (diabetes, autoimmune diseases, infections, and hereditary diseases)—will impair detoxification and will make the person far more susceptible to all chemical toxic substances.

It is for this reason that it is important to keep the liver healthy.

A Word about Pesticides, Herbicides, and Fungicides

The most commonly used pesticides are chemically classed as organophosphates, chlorinated hydrocarbons, or carbamates. These are very dangerous chemicals and should always be treated as such. Organophosphates are some of the mostly commonly used pesticides. They kill insects by inhibiting a specific enzyme that causes the insect's muscles to go haywire, rendering it unable to breath. Humans have the same enzyme, and a high enough dose of the pesticide can kill humans as well.

Yet, that is not the most dangerous thing about this class of pesticides. Researchers have found that this class of pesticides, as with all pesticides, herbicides, and fungicides, damage human cells at concentrations far lower than that known to inhibit the targeted enzyme. So, when companies insist that their product is safe because the levels of the chemical never get high enough to inhibit the targeted enzyme, this is just not so. Damage occurs at concentrations far below what would be expected and is done in completely different ways.

We are finding that these chemicals affect many of the processes the cell needs for normal functioning, and this makes us sick—very sick. Also, many of these chemicals are fat-soluble, meaning that they accumulate in our fat cells over our lifetime. Studies have shown that over 100 such chemicals can be found in the fat of most people. Overweight or obese people store the greatest amount of these chemicals. The brain, because it is 60% fat, also accumulates a great number of these toxic chemicals. A woman's breast tissue can store high concentrations of these chemicals, many of which are associated with breast cancer induction.

Because we are exposed to thousands of chemicals every day of our lives, over many years, we accumulate a high concentration of them in our fat cells. This is where it gets scary. If a chemically exposed person decides to lose weight, which is mainly fat weight, these chemicals are released from the fat cells into their blood stream and carried throughout their body. The faster we lose weight, the higher the concentration of these chemicals released. Our liver is also flooded with these newly released chemicals and must be in top shape to detoxify them. If our liver is healthy, we can detoxify most of these toxic chemicals and eliminate them from our body. If not, we will be poisoned worse than we were originally because these toxic substances will be released all at once in very high concentrations.

Under such a scenario, these toxic substances will be deposited in our organs (heart, lungs, spleen, liver, intestines, pancreas, etc.), and importantly, in our brain as it has a very high fat content.

Another unusual thing about pesticides and herbicides is that they are rapidly absorbed through our skin and enter the blood stream, quickly poisoning us. They are also rapidly absorbed if we inhale their fumes—not only into the lungs, but also into the olfactory nerves (smell nerves) traveling directly to critical areas of the brain. For this reason, you should avoid all chemical odors.

Many pesticides and herbicides have been banned based on unacceptable toxicity, especially as a link to carcinogenesis, that is, being able to cause cancer. While it is good that these chemicals have been banned, unfortunately many of these chemical agents will linger in the environment for decades, some much longer. For example, chlordane, a chlorinated cyclodiene (a type of insecticide), was banned in 1988, but not before 200 million pounds had been spread throughout homes and businesses. According to the EPA, more than 19 million homes were treated with chlordane before the ban went into effect, putting 52 million people at risk. Chlordane is a fat-soluble chemical that can persist in the body for many decades.

Chlordane, heptachlor, aldrin, endrin, and endosulfan, each with the same chemical classification, have all been used widely in homes and businesses. The irony is that several responsible scientists had been warning of the toxicity of these chemicals long before they were eventually banned. Makers of these harmful products used their financial influence to persuade Congress to hold off from banning them for as long as possible.

Banned, highly toxic and carcinogenic pesticides enter the U.S. in another way. Thanks to globalism, countries with stricter product controls buy food and products from countries with very lax controls, such as Mexico and Central American countries. Crops regularly treated with banned pesticides and herbicides are entering our food markets. Some of these banned agents are systemic pesticides, which cannot be washed off.

It is increasingly being recognized that some of the many breakdown products from pesticides, herbicides, and fungicides are equally toxic as the parent compound. These breakdown products are being found in hundreds of lakes, streams, ponds, and reservoirs.

Another concern with these agrichemicals is their effect on sexual development and sexual behavior, which is programmed in the brain early in life. Chlorpyrifos, a commonly used organophosphate pesticide used in homes, is particularly dangerous because it is lipid-soluble and can easily enter our cells, where it can do a great deal of damage, including to our DNA.

Studies have shown that exposure to this particular pesticide, early in life, can increase aggressive behavior in males, and sometimes cause hyperactivity as well. The exposures used in these studies were significantly less than were known to cause obvious toxicity. Several similar studies in animals have found that exposure soon after birth increased long-term behavioral changes, such as increased anxiety, which was worse in females. These pesticide-induced changes in behavior were caused by the abnormal development of brain pathways that control such behaviors.

Other pesticides are linked to a high incidence of cancer, especially lymphomas, which is increasing faster than any other type of cancer, especially among people in their 30s. From the late 1970s until 1992, there was a 50% increase in lymphomas, with the greatest incidence occurring in the farm belt of the Midwest.

The strongest links to cancer occurred with:

- Phenoxyacetic acids (especially 2,4-D)
- Organochlorines (chlordane, DDT, lindane, and toxaphene)
- Organophosphates such as diazinon, dichlorvos, and malathion

These are all commonly used pesticides—not only in commercial agriculture, but also in homes. You should be especially concerned about a pesticide called 2,4-D, which is commonly used in pasturelands, lawns, and golf courses, because it is strongly linked to non-Hodgkin's lymphoma.

Worst of all, these pesticides are causing cancers in doses far below those occurring in agriculture. In one recent study, for example, pesticide exposure was associated with a 71% increased risk of liver cancer, according to the meta-analysis, which was presented in 2019 at the American Association for Cancer Research's annual meeting in Washington, D.C.

Studies have shown that curcumin can protect the liver from damage caused by exposure to chlorpyrifos during pregnancy, increasing its ability to detoxify this harmful pesticide. Detoxification of these pesticides, herbicides, and fungicides is critical in protecting people from all these harmful effects.

Lindane, a now banned pesticide, has been shown to cause extensive damage to the liver because it produces high levels of free radicals and lipid peroxidation products and severely suppresses protective antioxidant enzymes and glutathione. By suppressing these antioxidant enzymes, lindane leaves the liver and other organs highly vulnerable to destruction and damage by free radicals and lipid peroxidation.

So, why would I mention a pesticide that has been banned? It has been estimated that 4.8 million tons of lindane is still present in the atmosphere as residue, as well as in soils. When it was approved for human use, lindane-containing shampoo was used to control head lice and scabies. This pesticide is rapidly absorbed through the lungs, the skin, and the gastrointestinal tract. Pesticides, such as lindane, when used within homes covers surfaces, including toys, and is easily absorbed via multiple routes.

In one study using mice exposed to lindane, it was shown that virtually all the damaging effects by lindane could be prevented and reversed by using curcumin orally. Curcumin was also shown to return all the antioxidant enzymes and glutathione to their normal protective levels. The beneficial effect was quite profound. Other studies found that a combination of vitamin C and vitamin E with curcumin was even more effective.

Glyphosate Herbicides: Contaminating the World

The herbicides containing the compound **glyphosate** are the most widely used weed killers in history. By 2014, the use of this toxic compound increased to 240 million pounds annually, just in the U.S. In 2000, the EPA announced that glyphosate was the "least toxic" herbicide in use. Further, they extended this deception by saying that glyphosate-type herbicides do not bioaccumulate, they do not contaminate the ground water, have no toxic effects on animals, don't cause cancer, and are quickly eliminated from the environment once dispersed. Extensive independent studies demonstrate that none of these assurances are true.

Instead, it was discovered that these plants quickly became resistant to the weed killer, which led farmers to use progressively increasing amounts of this herbicide on their crops. In an effort to allow farmers greater use of weed killers at higher concentrations, one company genetically engineered certain crops, such as soybeans (called Roundup Ready soybeans), to be highly resistant to its weed killer. This would allow farmers to control weeds without harming their crops. The company could then sell its special Roundup-resistant seeds each season, as well as sell a lot more weed killer. Studies have found much higher concentrations of this herbicide in these crops. Unlike pesticides that are used mainly for commercial agriculture, weed killer use extends to millions of homes, golf courses, and public facilities.

Because these herbicides do indeed bioaccumulate—that is, linger with each application, leading to higher and higher concentrations in the environment—levels were quickly being reached that were known to be toxic, in many ways, to virtually every living animal, from one-cell organisms to humans.

Most studies showing they were safe, were conducted by individuals and firms with a financial interest in the companies making these chemicals. One deception by the makers was to conduct studies that only tested the main ingredient—**glyphosate**, and not the actual products being used, such as Roundup. They did this because they knew glyphosate had a lower level of toxicity than did the whole product and that glyphosate alone was poorly absorbed. All the herbicide products using glyphosate combine this main ingredient with what is called a **surfactant** or **adjuvant**, which dramatically increases absorption of the herbicide through the skin, and in addition increases absorption when ingested or inhaled. These special additives also contribute a separate toxicity of their own that is even greater than the main ingredient, glyphosate. Together, the whole product constitutes a major environmental toxic hazard.

Studies using rats demonstrated that this weed killer caused severe histopathological damage to the liver, with degeneration of cells in the liver and kidneys along with infiltration of the liver with macrophage immune cells. This causes further, long-term damage to the liver. In one study, researchers examined the level of glyphosate in individuals with NAFLD and NASH and found that those with evidence of liver fibrosis and NASH (advanced nonalcoholic steatohepatitis) had significantly higher levels of glyphosate and its chief metabolite, AMPA, in their urine, as compared to those with NAFLD or normal liver function. Other studies have shown that the weed killer causes a significant decline in sperm cells and a greatly increased number of abnormal sperm cells.

Several studies have shown that glyphosate is a potent endocrine disrupter, causing interference with both male and female sexual development, as well as alterations in sexual function later in life. The doses used in this extensive study were at levels accepted by the EPA as safe for human exposure. In fact, studies have shown that endocrine disruption by glyphosate occurs at doses that are **800 times lower** than the concentration recommended by the EPA as safe for food contamination. This herbicide has also been shown to interfere with the liver's detoxification function, meaning that it puts a person at extreme risk even from exposure to otherwise mild toxic substances.

The greatest amount of Roundup used is in treating soybean plants. Studies have shown that Roundup residues are found in 90% of soybean products, the majority of which are GMO.

Another study found that Roundup, and other such herbicides, induced estrogen-sensitive breast cancer cell proliferation by stimulating estrogen receptors on breast cancer cells. Again, very low concentrations of glyphosate were used in this study. The highest concentration of glyphosate herbicides is used in treating soybean fields. Ironically, soybeans also contain a naturally occurring estrogenic compound called **genistein**, which means that all products made from these treated soybean products are heavily contaminated with two endocrine disrupting compounds—**genistein** and **glyphosate**. This includes soybean milk, soybean-based baby formula, soybean food additives, soy cheeses, and numerous other soybean products.

Massive amounts of glyphosate-containing herbicides are being used on crops, especially in the U.S. There is increasing concern of contamination of public drinking water with these herbicides, as well as extensive contamination of foods, including vegetables, sugar, wheat, beef, and pork, and hundreds of other commonly used products, including vaccines, medications, and breads.

Recent studies have also shown that crop fields treated repeatedly with Roundup and similar herbicides, produced vegetables of lower nutrient content and farmers experienced lower crop yields.

Roundup is one of the more popular herbicides being used in suburbs and cities as well. Most of these extremely toxic compounds are being stored in garages attached to houses. Spills and leaks are common, which means vapors not only accumulate in the garage, but also the house as well. Children are at an even greater risk than adults.

Other Endocrine Disrupters and Toxic Substances

While pesticides, herbicides, and fungicides constitute a major source of endocrine disrupters, there are many others hidden in our everyday world. Included among these commonly used industrial chemicals are polychlorinated biphenyls (PCBs), dioxins, pesticides, herbicides, phthalates, and bisphenol A. These are highly reactive chemicals that tend to persist in the environment, bioaccumulate, and alter endocrine function, leading to a number of disorders.

Phthalates are a class of industrial chemicals that have contaminated a great deal of our environment. It has been determined that 100% of the U.S. population has some level of one or more of these compounds in their tissues. Phthalates have contaminated indoor and outdoor dust, foods, milk, and drinking water.

The high molecular weight forms, (DEHP) diethylhexyl phthalates, are used as plasticizers in manufacturing polyvinyl chloride (PVC), which is employed in wall coverings, the lining for cans of food and drinks, and medical devices. The lower molecular forms are used as industrial solvents and plasticizers for cellulose acetate in making lacquers, varnishes, coatings, and some personal care products (perfumes, lotions, and cosmetics).

One of the truly frightening effects of phthalates is the ability of these compounds to act as anti-androgens (blocks male hormone). Using a special technique to determine development of sexual organs, researchers found that there was a very strong link between exposure to phthalates during pregnancy and development of male sexual organs, but not female sexual organs. The doses causing the problem were relatively low. Numerous animal studies have shown these same types of effects.

The study was one of the largest ever done, involving 737 infants (365 males and 372 females). For the study, they measured the level of phthalates in the urine of the babies. In the animal studies, researchers found a link to abnormal development of the male reproductive organs, which included:

- Incomplete descent of testes
- Smaller testes and penis
- Alteration in the vas deferens and epididymis

In human babies, we see such abnormal reproductive disorders as hypospadias, cryptorchidism, smaller penis, poor sperm quality, and reduced levels of testosterone. These defects in male reproductive organs and sperm occurred when the exposure happened during the first trimester of pregnancy.

Another study of older children found that those exposed to phthalates during pregnancy exhibited reduced masculine play—that is, they were not acting like typical boys. The mothers of the affected children were found to have the highest levels of phthalates in their urine during pregnancy with the child. They concluded that these chemicals caused an abnormal development of the brain structures responsible for male behavior. Specific types of phthalates were involved. The more of these that were involved, the greater the impact on male behavior.

Fortunately, the concentration of phthalates found in the environment has fallen considerably.

Another ubiquitous environmental chemical of concern is bisphenol A (BPA), which is a synthetic chemical used in the manufacture of polycarbonate plastics and epoxy resins. BPA is one of the most widely used synthetic compounds on the planet, with an annual production of 5 million tons in the U.S. alone. Exposure to BPA occurs mostly through contaminated canned foods. While canned food is a significant source of BPA contamination, by far the greatest exposure is from thermal receipts used to check you out of a store or restaurant. If your fingers are wet or greasy, the levels are 10 times higher than if dry and if you use a hand sanitizer, absorption through the skin is even higher because most such products contain a compound to increase skin absorption.

Studies have shown that BPA residues are found in about 93% of people examined.

A study of pregnant women found that the highest concentration is in the placenta and the fetus. This is of major concern because BPA can cause birth defects and has been associated with a high incidence of repeated miscarriages. BPA has been found in breast milk.

The liver can detoxify BPA by two processes that can eliminate the toxic product in the urine. Unfortunately, BPA also damages the liver, thus impairing its own detoxification. BPA reduces the liver's antioxidant enzymes, which allows the chemical to severely damage the liver cells involved in detoxification. It also causes severe DNA damage in liver cells.

This compound can also activate brain microglia, which causes inflammation of the brain and prolonged destruction of brain cells (neurodegeneration). Another finding of concern is that BPA was found to cause DNA damage in breast cancer cells and stimulate faster cancer growth.

One of the major environmental pollutants is polychlorinated biphenyls (PCBs), a chemical introduced for large scale use in 1945, with 1.3 million tons being manufactured before it was banned in 1979. They were not banned until 1990 in some other countries. Unfortunately, PCBs are resistant to degradation and therefore continue to persist all over the world. They accumulate in the bottoms of rivers, ponds, lakes, and seas, contaminating bottom-feeding creatures. Fish are contaminated with PCBs all over the world.

What makes this chemical so dangerous to people is that it is fat soluble, meaning it can accumulate in the body's fat deposits for a lifetime. This leads to chronic inflammation and continuous generation of free radicals and lipid peroxidation. As a result, a number of diseases are linked to PCB exposure, including obesity, cardiovascular diseases, strokes, hypertension, heart attacks, and cancers of the liver, stomach, intestines, and thyroid, and non-Hodgkin's lymphoma.

PCBs are also associated with reproductive abnormalities, diabetes, insulin resistance, metabolic syndrome, impaired thyroid function, reduced immunity, and an assortment of liver diseases, such as NAFLD, NASH, and liver cancer. Because PCBs cause chronic inflammation, one's health can progressively deteriorate over time. And because PCBs mainly attack the liver, detoxification of other poisons and toxic compounds is also impaired.

Fluoride and Fluoroaluminum Complexes

Fluoride and aluminum are both commonly found in our environment and unfortunately are used in many products and dental treatments. Drinking water is a major source of both of these elements. In all their wisdom, city governments, and even governors of states, have mandated the addition of fluoride and aluminum to public drinking water systems.

A massive propaganda effort, based on no scientific evidence, convinced the dental profession and public health officials that fluoride added to drinking water would drastically reduce dental cavities. Every major study told an opposite story. Rather than reducing dental cavity incidence, the fluoride was actually weakening the dental enamel, subjecting the teeth to more risk of cavities and discolored teeth, a condition called *dental fluorosis*. The incidence of dental fluorosis increased drastically following fluoridation of drinking water.

A great number of studies confirmed that not only was fluoride ineffective at preventing cavities, but fluoridation of drinking water was associated with many serious conditions, including the induction of rare cancers, stimulation of the spread of other cancers, the lowering of children's IQ, the weakening of bones with a resulting increase in spontaneous fractures (especially in women), damage to brain structures, reduced thyroid function, and DNA damage.

Most cities add 1 to 1.5 ppm (parts per million) to drinking water. Of major concern is that fluoride accumulates in tissues, especially in critical brain structures, such as the hippocampus and pineal gland, causing significant damage. Bone also accumulates very high levels of fluoride, as high as thousands of ppm. This severely weakens the bones, which are then subject to spontaneous stress fractures, especially to the hip and bones of the forearms.

In truth, the fluoride in drinking water combines with the added aluminum forming what is called a **fluoroaluminum complex**, which is very destructive. In fact, fluoroaluminum in a concentration half that of fluoride alone (0.5ppm) can cause considerable tissue and organ damage. Both fluoride and aluminum are found in many foods and drinks. Black tea contains very high levels of both metals. Grapes, raisins, spinach, sodas, coffee, and shrimp all contain rather high levels of fluoride, but in most cases this fluoride is in a less toxic form than is being added to public drinking water.

Aluminum is one of the most abundant elements found on earth. Teas are usually the number one source of aluminum in foodstuffs, but all canned foods in aluminum cans are at risk. Most cans are lined with a coating (usually BPA-containing), but breaks in these linings allow leaching of the aluminum from the container. Acidic foods and drinks leach the greatest amount of aluminum from cans.

Other sources of aluminum include all aluminum cookware, any food using baking powder (in virtually all biscuits), aluminum foil, aluminum trays, and aluminum cups.

Because aluminum and fluoride are both highly reactive chemicals, wherever they occur together they rapidly combine to form the highly destructive fluoroaluminum complex. There is a strong connection between aluminum in the nervous system and several neurological disorders, such as Alzheimer's disease and ALS.

Because all aluminum products primarily enter the body by way of the gastrointestinal system, the first target for toxicity is the liver. Fluoroaluminum poisons all types of liver cells, especially the ones used in detoxification. Again, this makes a person highly susceptible to all toxic substances. Aluminum alone is poorly absorbed from the GI tract, but as a fluoroaluminum complex it is better absorbed.

One of the main sources of aluminum is vaccines. Aluminum is used in most vaccines as an immune booster (adjuvant). Unlike oral aluminum exposures, 100% of injected aluminum from vaccines is absorbed and rapidly distributed to all areas of the body, including the brain. This absorbed aluminum is stored in the body for very long periods, even for a lifetime. Each dose (or vaccine) adds considerably to the total burden of aluminum in the tissues and organs.

In a 2019 study, researchers found that fluoride exposure may lead to a reduction in kidney and liver function in adolescents. While fluoride exposure in animals and adults has been associated with kidney and liver toxicity, this study examined potential effects of chronic, low-level exposure among youth.

The researchers say this was an important study because a child's body excretes only 45% of fluoride in the urine via the kidneys, while an adult's body clears it at a rate of 60%, and the kidneys accumulate more fluoride than any other organ in the body. While fluoride exposure in animals and adults has been associated with kidney and liver toxicity, this study examined the potential effects of chronic, low-level exposure among youths, which could cause even greater damage.

Fluoride is also used to enhance the length of time prescription drugs remain in the body, mainly by inhibiting the liver's detoxification enzymes. Adding fluoride to medications also greatly increases their toxicity. Many of these drugs are associated with very dangerous side effects, including suicidal thoughts and even homicidal thoughts. They also cause severe damage to the liver and kidneys. Many of the newer antibiotics contain fluoride. The major SSRI psychotropic medications are also fluoridated.

Another source of fluoride is from polyfluorinated chemicals (PFCs), which are used in various industrial processes and consumer products because of their property of repelling dirt, water, and oils. The most commonly used include perfluorooctane sulfonic acid (PFOS) and perfluorooctanoic acid (PFOA), both of which persist in the environment for very long periods. These compounds have been detected in air, water, soil, and wildlife—even in the polar regions.

In humans, these products accumulate in tissues over time. While these compounds were banned in 2000, they continue to persist in the environment. Hundreds of related chemicals continue to be used and are not regulated. Animal studies have shown that these chemicals can cause liver and kidney damage of a substantial nature. The highest bioaccumulation was in the liver, with progressively less in the heart, kidney, lungs, and brain. Some animal studies have shown that these chemicals can cause cancer, damage reproductive organs, cause brain damage, and are toxic to the liver.

It is important to avoid as many chemical agents as possible, and when working with these compounds, one should wear a respirator mask and use high-speed room ventilation or at least be in a well-ventilated space.

The safest teas to drink are white tea or green tea. Both have much lower levels of fluoride and aluminum, but white tea is the best. These two teas also have flavonoids that protect the liver and other organs from toxicity by these chemicals.

One should also eat only organically grown or raised foods. It is important to choose healthy organic vegetables, because damaged or moldy vegetables contain natural carcinogenic substances that the plant uses to protect itself. All water should be filtered or distilled. I prefer distilled water, which I add magnesium to after distilling.

Other Chemicals

Chemicals you may be exposed to on the job can cause liver injury, and this includes white collar jobs. Most businesses use a pesticide service, which sprays toxic pesticides in each private office and in common areas, including break rooms. Common chemicals, which can be toxic to the liver (and hence are known as hepatoxins) include the dry-cleaning solvent carbon tetrachloride, a substance called *vinyl chloride* (used to make plastics), and many other industrial chemicals employed in manufacturing.

Work activities involving hepatotoxin exposure are numerous and include chemists, dry cleaners, farmworkers, painters, health care workers, landscaping businesses, plant nurseries, businesses selling pesticides, herbicides, and fungicides, gardeners, home pesticide workers, termite company employees, hospital employees and patients, and printers. Organic solvents are used in various industrial processes, such as spray painting, paint manufacturing, degreasing, metal processing, aeronautical and auto manufacturing, maintenance and manufacturing, as well as various chemical storage facilities. Welders are exposed to several toxic metal vapors.

Exposure to hepatotoxins can occur through accidents, garage contamination, ingestion of foods or drinks, or absorption of toxic contaminants through the skin. Contamination includes the ingestion of public drinking water, skin absorption via water baths, swimming in polluted waters, and volatilization of solvents and paints.

While most deaths occur from acute exposures, such as farm accidents where a person falls in a vat of pesticides or herbicides, most poisonings are occurring chronically and the victim may be completely unaware of it, because most of these agents are in concentrations that have no odor or taste. Living near a manufacturing plant or a farm can expose one to airborne toxic substances carried by the winds. Contaminated ground water and runoff from surface pollutants pose a danger to public drinking water.

Children are at far greater risk from these toxic substances than adults because of body size and differences in their metabolism and detoxification ability. Playing sports on a field in which glyphosate-containing weed killers, such as Roundup, are used poses a major danger for neurotoxicity and cancer development, especially for lymphomas, multiple myelomas, and leukemias.

Protecting Your Liver

Fortunately, there are a number of things one can do to protect the liver from these toxic substances and enhance one's detoxification ability. For example, saffron has shown an ability to reduce the toxicity of organophosphate pesticides. Saffron has antico-agulant properties, so it should not be used in combination with other anticoagulants.

Taurine and Nano-Curcumin enhance the detoxification of chlorpyrifos and rotenone. Rotenone is widely used to kill unwanted fish species in lakes and ponds, but it is strongly linked to Parkinson's disease. In fact, it is used in experimental animals to induce a Parkinson's-like disorder. Other things that reduce rotenone toxicity include blueberry extract, Nano-Grape Seed extract, and Nano-Curcumin. The triple plant extract Triphala reduces chlorpyrifos toxicity.

While these natural compounds are directed at specific pesti-cides, other compounds are also powerful general liver protectants against all such liver toxins. The most important include Nano-Curcumin, Nano-Grape Seed extract, Nano-Silymarin, vitamin E (as mixed tocopherols), mixed tocotrienols, Nano-Vitamin C, hesperidin, apigenin, luteolin, L-carnitine, and baicalin. In fact, baicalin shows quite potent liver protecting effects among these compounds, and a combination of Nano-Curcumin and baicalin is even more effective. One study, on people with liver fibrosis, the stage just before liver cirrhosis, demonstrated a significant reduc-tion in liver fibrosis when taking baicalin long term.

Another of the leaders in liver protection, especially in preventing and treating nonalcoholic fatty liver disease (NAFLD) and NASH, the more advanced form of the disease, is **L-carnitine**. Several carefully conducted human studies have shown this natural compound dramatically reduced fatty liver disease and just as dramatically reduced visceral fat as well. One of the major problems seen with patients with liver cirrhosis is a loss of muscle mass. L-carnitine has been shown to suppress the loss of muscle in patients with cirrhosis.

As liver destruction advances, patients will experience a number of neurological problems affecting mentation and alertness, a condition called **hepatic encephalopathy**. L-carnitine has been shown to significantly protect advanced cirrhotic patients from intellectual loss and confusion.

Any natural compound that can reduce inflammation and free radical/lipid peroxidation will reduce the damage produced by these chemical agents. Other beneficial compounds include R-lipoic acid, N-acetyl-L-cysteine (NAC), B-complex vitamins, myo-inositol, trans-ferulic acid, and pterostilbene. Pterostilbene, which is converted to resveratrol once absorbed, has been shown to protect against fatty liver disease. Pterostilbene is absorbed about four times better than resveratrol.

Studies using taurine, a sulfur-containing amino acid, demonstrate powerful protection against NAFLD and other liver injuries. One study demonstrated powerful effects by taurine supplementation in preventing liver fibrosis, the stage before liver cirrhosis develops.

CHAPTER 9

How Drugs Can
Poison Your Liver

The drugs you take may benefit your body, but at the same time, they can damage your liver because one of your liver's main jobs is to metabolize them. According to carefully done studies, anywhere from 100,000 to 300,000 people die each year from drug reactions, excluding allergic reactions and overdoses.

Your body has a way of dealing with drugs you take, and it is a four-step process known as "ADME," an acronym that stands for absorption, distribution, metabolism, and excretion.

Medicines are absorbed when they travel from the site of administration into the body's circulation. This can be through many ways, such as by mouth or injection, or done intravenously, to name just a few. Once a drug gets absorbed, it travels, usually through the bloodstream, to the location that is its target.

Drugs taken by mouth are first carried to the liver, where most are metabolized, and some are changed into other compounds. Drugs that are absorbed through the skin or injected reach the liver after they have circulated throughout the body.

Keep in mind that all cells have a detoxification system that also metabolizes these drugs.

In the liver, the absorbed substances are often chemically altered and transformed by enzymes. However, some are not detoxified, and instead are altered by other metabolic processes in the liver. This is true not only of medications, but also of herbal products and supplements. For some drugs, the liver detoxifies the compound via the phase I and phase II processes discussed in Chapter 1, ultimately removing the drug from the body either by the bile through the feces or by way of the kidneys.

For some products, another problem arises—the drug may directly harm the liver's cells, impairing the liver's function. This condition is known as liver toxicity, hepatic toxicity, or toxic hepatitis, which means that, under such circumstances, the liver has impaired detoxification and metabolizing ability. When this happens, the toxicity of drugs increases substantially. Should this occur, drugs that normally would be safe become dangerous, even in prescribed doses. Depending on the product, medications, chemicals, solvents, alcohol, herbal supplements, and chemotherapy can all cause liver toxicity. Pharmaceutical drugs have been shown to be far more harmful than natural substances. Deaths caused by natural products are rather rare, unlike pharmaceutical drugs.

Damage to the liver can vary substantially, from a mild elevation of liver enzymes to acute liver failure. Most mild to moderate liver damage is 100% reversible. In cases of acute liver failure, the outcome depends on the toxic substance one is exposed to. In cases of acetaminophen poisoning, for example, most people, even with acute liver failure, if treated early, will completely recover. With other substances, the liver does not recover, and the person develops what is called **hepatic encephalopathy**, which ends in coma and death rather rapidly. Some 2000 cases of liver failure occur each year, which are directly due to the effects of medications.

Sometimes medications are life-saving and cannot be avoided, but too often, liver damage can occur because too much medication is unthinkingly consumed (combining two or more liver toxic substances), the medication is extremely liver toxic, or the person has an undiagnosed preexisting liver impairment.

The liver has one of the most remarkable abilities to regenerate of all the organs and tissues in the body. Even extensive damage to the liver can often be repaired, especially if special antioxidants and anti-inflammatory natural compounds are given.

The following factors raise your risk of toxic liver disease:

- Being age 65 or older
- Being female
- Taking more over-the-counter pain relievers than the recommended dose
- Taking over-the-counter pain relievers, or certain medications or supplements with alcohol
- Combining one or more liver toxic substances at the same time (drug synergy)
- Chronic use of artificial sweeteners that are known to be liver toxic, such as aspartame
- Having an underlying liver condition, such as cirrhosis, fatty liver disease, or hepatitis
- Working or having worked in a job that uses industrial chemicals that can damage the liver
- Having a genetic mutation that affects the liver's detoxification function

Symptoms of Toxic Liver Disease

- Unexplained fever
- Diarrhea

- Dark-colored urine
- Itching
- Jaundice, or yellowish eyes and skin
- Headaches
- Loss of appetite
- Nausea
- Stomach pain or pain on the upper right-hand side of the abdomen
- Vomiting
- Weight loss
- White or gray stool

Some Drugs that Cause Liver Toxicity

- Acetaminophen (Tylenol)
- Amoxicillin/clavulanate (Augmentin)
- Diclofenac (Voltaren, Cambia)
- Amiodarone (Cordarone, Pacerone)
- Allopurinol (Zyloprim)
- Antiseizure medications
- Methotrexate
- Statins (cholesterol-lowering medication)
- Antipsychotic medications

Acetaminophen (Tylenol)

Acetaminophen works well as a fever reducer and pain reliever but is one of the most common causes of acute liver failure in the United States and United Kingdom. Of the acute liver failure cases attributed to medications, an estimated one-half are due to acetaminophen. Acetaminophen overdoses account for 20% of liver transplants and result in 450 deaths annually. In the U.S., acetaminophen accounts for 26,000 hospital admissions each year.

Many cases of acetaminophen-related acute liver failure are linked to suicide attempts, yet in up to 61 to 79% of cases the poisoning was unintentional. Almost 80% of such cases occur in women. Mortality and morbidity are more common with unintentional poisoning than intentional incidents, mainly because most unintentional cases are caused by errors in judgment or taking two or more medications with acetaminophen as an ingredient.

An unknown number of cases are caused by doses near or even at recommended doses, when we take other factors into consideration. For example, chronic use of alcohol can deplete glutathione levels, the main liver detoxification system for this drug. Other drugs and medical conditions, even fasting or starvation dieting, can deplete liver glutathione levels, thus increasing the vulnerability to acetaminophen poisoning. Many chronic diseases can deplete liver glutathione levels, such as steatohepatitis (NASH). Older people (over age 40) have a greater vulnerability to acetaminophen toxicity.

One product that causes severe depletion of hepatic glutathione is the artificial sweetener aspartame, the regular use of which can make one much more sensitive to acetaminophen toxicity, because glutathione is the main detoxification system for the acetaminophen by-product causing the liver damage (called NAPQI). Many people are addicted to aspartame, which can make them highly susceptible to acetaminophen liver and kidney damage, even with approved dosages.

Symptoms of acetaminophen poisoning usually begin within 24 hours and go through four phases, ending in acute liver failure. Most people, if treated, will recover from acetaminophen poisoning, even with liver failure. If not treated, this form of poisoning can lead to rapid death or the need for a liver transplant.

Like many drugs, acetaminophen is metabolized in the liver. Most of it gets broken down and altered into substances that are uneventfully excreted in the urine.

In most cases, acetaminophen is mostly metabolized into relatively harmless compounds, but it will produce a small amount of the harmful product NAPQI. Usually, NAPQI is rendered harmless because it combines with glutathione in the liver cells. However, if there's too much NAPQI, which can happen with an acetaminophen overdose, or when liver glutathione levels are low prior to the drug exposure, liver damage can occur. High levels of this metabolic product can severely deplete glutathione levels.

More than 600 products contain acetaminophen, and most cases of liver damage occur from accidentally combining them, because many drugs use acetaminophen as an ingredient. This practice is also common with prescription drugs.

Treatment of liver damage by acetaminophen is usually dependent on taking N-acetyl-L-cysteine, which rapidly raises glutathione levels. The best results are when NAC is taken within 16 hours of the drug exposure. While most people can take NAC orally, some are allergic to the sulfur component (cysteine) in NAC. In very rare cases, these allergic reactions can be fatal.

Fortunately, there are other natural compounds that can inhibit acetaminophen liver damage just as well as NAC, such as Nano-Curcumin, Nano-Quercetin, Nano-Silymarin, apigenin, luteolin, berberine, hesperidin, baicalin, vitamins C and E, and trans-ferulic acid. A number of these compounds can restore damaged liver function, as well as restore suppressed antioxidant enzymes and glutathione.

A recent study found that curcumin works just as well as NAC, and at higher doses, even better, in that all the toxic effects on the liver were shown to be completely reversed to normal, including the elevated enzymes, high-level lipid peroxidation, and histological damage. Acetaminophen also damages the kidneys. This same study found that curcumin could also reverse all the damage to the kidneys as well. Combining curcumin to a much lower dose of NAC was also successful in reversing the liver and kidney damage.

Nano-Curcumin is absorbed much better and is more effective than other formulations of curcumin. The best results are obtained when the Nano-Curcumin is given within 24 hours of the acetaminophen overdose. The sooner the better. The Nano-Curcumin can be continued permanently for at least a month. The dose would be 500 mg taken three times a day with food.

Another recent study found that silymarin also effectively protected the liver and kidneys from acetaminophen damage. In this study, silymarin given after the acetaminophen returned liver enzymes, antioxidant levels, BUN and creatinine, glutathione, and the histology of these two organs to normal. In the kidney, elevated nitric oxide caused by the acetaminophen, a sign of kidney damage, was also returned to normal. The important thing about silymarin is that it not only stopped the damage; it actively reversed and repaired the damage by promoting protein synthesis. Nano-Silymarin is significantly better absorbed than other formulations of silymarin. The dose is 500 mg taken three times a day with meals.

Because of the potential damage caused by even accepted doses of acetaminophen, I would never promote its use under any condition. There are a great number of natural compounds that relieve pain and lower an elevated temperature that are far safer. In general, fever should not be lowered (unless extreme) in cases of infections (especially viral infections) because the fever helps kill the infectious organisms. Studies have shown that lowering the fever in children with viral illnesses dramatically raises the mortality of the infection.

Antibiotics

Antibiotics, as with most drugs taken by mouth, are exposed first to the liver after absorption, where they are metabolized. Keep in mind that all tissues can metabolize drugs, but the liver is the main site of detoxification and metabolism. Once metabolized, the antibiotic is neutralized and excreted from the body. This is why antibiotics are given on a regular schedule—that is, to keep blood levels high so they can cure the infection. For example, penicillin may be given every 6 hours. Toward the end of the sixth hour, so much of the drug has been neutralized by the detoxification process that little is left to treat the infection. So, another dose must be given just before that occurs.

Things that interfere with the detoxification of these drugs will allow the drug to remain at high blood levels longer. Many natural products can interfere with the phase I detoxification of these drugs. Pharmacists have tables that inform them of such interactions with natural compounds. This explains why you should always tell your doctor what natural compounds you are taking.

Patients with liver diseases, such as cirrhosis, have impaired drug detoxification, meaning that many drugs will stay in the blood longer than normal, raising the risk of an overdose even when taking the drugs as prescribed.

Some antibiotics have a direct toxicity on the liver. Antibiotics most often implicated with liver injury are amoxicillin/clavulanic acid, flucloxacillin, azithromycin, chloramphenicol, lincomycin, and erythromycin.

Newer antibiotics contain a fluorine compound within their chemical structure, which is designed to suppress detoxification, allowing the drug to remain in a higher concentration longer. We call these antibiotics fluoroquinolones, and they include ciprofloxacin (Cipro), gemifloxacin (Factive), levofloxacin (Levaquin), moxifloxacin (Avelox), norfloxacin (Noroxin), and ofloxacin (Floxin).

Fluoridated antibiotics such as these have a significantly higher complication rate, and like most fluoridated drugs, they can be associated with suicidal thoughts and homicidal ideation. This class of fluorine-containing drugs are more difficult for the body to detoxify. Some of these drugs will release their fluorine, which can cause severe toxicity itself.

Arthritis Drugs

Methotrexate and azathioprine are the drugs most often associated with liver damage. Methotrexate slows the progression of rheumatoid arthritis (RA) and relieves symptoms by causing cells to release a molecule called *adenosine*, which blocks other chemicals that promote inflammation. According to the Arthritis Foundation, liver damage secondary to methotrexate use occurs in 1 out of every 1000 people, and your doctor may recommend you avoid alcohol and undergo blood tests to monitor your liver.

Next to antibiotics, non-steroidal anti-inflammatory drugs (NSAIDs) are the second-most common cause of drug-induced liver injury. Fatty liver diseases (NAFLD and NASH) and metabolic syndrome can weaken the liver, making NSAIDs even more liver toxic. The same is true for alcohol abuse, and the use of acetaminophen and aspartame. It has also been determined that patients taking other liver toxic medications are six to nine times more susceptible to liver damage by NSAIDs. These would include antibiotics, proton-pump inhibitors (ulcer medications), aspartame, phenobarbital, halothane (an anesthetic), and isoniazid (a TB medication).

Autoimmune diseases, such as rheumatoid arthritis, cause liver damage themselves, which makes the liver more vulnerable to all medications used to treat the condition. In the past, severe cases of rheumatoid arthritis required higher doses of several medications known to cause liver toxicity.

Aspirin can cause some liver damage if used in higher doses for a prolonged period, especially in rheumatoid arthritis. Sulindac has a higher incidence of liver damage than other arthritis medications such as diclofenac and especially ibuprofen, which have a very low incidence of liver toxicity and kidney damage. Again, when combined with other liver toxic compounds and in conditions associated with liver impairment, even low-toxicity drugs can become quite toxic.

There are a great many anti-inflammatory natural compounds that not only do not damage the liver or kidneys; they are powerful liver protectants, such as Nano-Curcumin, Nano-Silymarin, L-carnitine, and baicalin. When combined with pharmaceutical drugs for arthritis, these natural anti-inflammatory compounds enhance the effectiveness and safety of the drugs.

Antifungal Drugs

Antifungal drugs can damage the liver. Because of this, your doctor should monitor your liver functions, particularly if you have an underlying liver disease. Liver toxicity of these medications varies widely with the type of medication used. Most antifungal medications carry a warning to reduce the dosage in patients with known liver problems, yet for most antifungal medications, liver toxicity is minimal and resolves with discontinuation of the drug.

Flucytosine, a fluorine-containing drug, can cause liver damage by stimulating inflammation, but its most toxic effects are directed at the bone marrow. The azole class of antifungals, which includes ketoconazole, miconazole, and clotrimazole, generally cause mild liver damage, but cases of fatal liver failure have been described. Micafungin is metabolized in the liver by enzymes other than P-450 phase I enzymes, but it carries a warning concerning use in patients with liver diseases and has a possible link to liver tumors. Voriconazole can cause severe liver injury in patients with preexisting liver impairment.

Niacin

Niacin can be used to lower cholesterol, but should not be taken in large doses, especially if you have an underlying liver disease. Another formulation of niacin, inositol hexanicotinate (also known as inositol hexaniacinate), does not cause liver damage. Niacinamide is thought to have little toxic effects on the liver, but higher doses, especially in those with preexisting liver impairment, create a higher risk of liver damage. Niacinamide in megadoses (several grams a day) have been associated with occasional cases of liver toxicity of a milder degree. In general, it is preferable to use doses of no more than 2 to 3 grams a day. It has been used to treat osteoarthritis, type 1 diabetes, and schizophrenia with some success. Higher doses have been used to enhance the beneficial effects of radiation treatment of cancers.

Steroids

Corticosteroids also have a major effect on the liver, particularly when given long term and in higher than recommended doses, and can trigger or worsen NASH, the more serious form of fatty liver disease. Glucocorticoid use can result in liver enlargement and fat storage in the liver. Yet, these drugs have been used to treat liver failure associated with viral hepatitis and autoimmune liver disease with great success. When used for such conditions, most often in the short term, corticosteroids can be lifesaving.

Amiodarone (Cordarone, Pacerone)

This cardiovascular drug used to treat arrhythmias, or irregular heartbeats, can cause liver damage in up to 1% of users, usually at higher doses and/or with prolonged use.

Allopurinol (Zyloprim)

Part of a drug class called *xanthine oxidase inhibitors*, allopurinol, which is used to treat gout, can cause liver failure in rare cases.

Antiseizure Medications

Several anti-epileptic medications can cause liver damage. Dilantin (phenytoin) can cause problems shortly after it is begun, which is why liver monitoring is done, and carbamazepine and lamotrigine can cause liver problems that can show up later. If you need epilepsy drugs, you should discuss this with your doctor. There are other anti-epileptic drugs that are considered safer for the liver. In fact, most seizures can be controlled with a change in diet and use of anti-inflammatory and anti–free radical natural products. I have used these natural compounds with great success. The real advantage is that they not only stop most seizures; they also improve general health, including liver health. These include Nano-Curcumin, Nano-Ashwagandha, taurine, baicalin, Nano-Bacopa, myoinositol, and magnesium.

Psychotropic Medications

These are drugs that are used as antidepressants, mood stabilizers, antianxiety, and antipsychotics, and many have the potential to cause liver damage. Other psychotropic drugs associated with a high incidence of liver injury include the tricyclic antidepressants—imipramine, amitriptyline, venlafaxine, duloxe-tine, sertraline, and bupropion. A rather long list of antipsychotic medications are also hepatotoxic, which includes chlorpromazine, haloperidol, clozapine, risperidone, and ziprasidone.

Among the mood stabilizers, lamotrigine, valproate, topira-mate, and carbamazepine are all associated with occasional liver injury, especially in those individuals with preexisting liver dis-orders. In most cases, the effect is limited to simple elevations in liver enzymes, which reverse when the mediations are either stopped or the dose is reduced.

Statins

One of the liver's most important functions is to produce and regulate cholesterol distribution in the body. Cholesterol is essen-tial for a number of physiological functions in the body and is used extensively by the brain. Marketing statin cholesterol low-ering drugs was based on the fallacious idea that elevated choles-terol itself was the cause of atherosclerosis and therefore linked to heart attacks and strokes. This has been disproven, and once the patent ran out on this class of drugs, cardiologists began to admit that the statin drugs had been oversold. New studies have clearly demonstrated that inflammation is the cause of atherosclerosis and that only a single class of oxidized cholesterol (small dense LDL-cholesterol) poses any risk to people. The strongest link is to excess omega-6 oils in the diet and sugar.

Statins include atorvastatin (Lipitor), fluvastatin (Lescol XL), lovastatin (Altoprev), pitavastatin (Livalo), pravastatin (Pravachol), rosuvastatin (Crestor, Ezallor), and simvastatin (Zocor, FloLipid). Statins are associated with liver injury and muscle injury in a dose-related way, meaning the higher the dose, the more likely injury to these two tissues could occur. Statins deplete Coenzyme Q10 production by inhibiting the same enzyme used in cholesterol production. Severe, often irreversible damage to skeletal muscles are common with the use of these drugs.

As greater use of statins began after their introduction, more cases of liver and muscle injury were being reported. Rosuvastatin has been shown to cause a higher incidence of liver injury than other statins, mainly because hepatocytes, the main cells of the liver, take up this drug in much higher concentrations than other statins. In addition, all statins, except simvastatin, worsened insulin resistance, a major process in liver disorders, as well as Alzheimer's disease, atherosclerosis, and cardiovascular diseases.

CHAPTER 10

Your Adrenal Gland and Your Liver

A gland is an organ that secretes chemicals that the body needs for functioning. The small, triangular adrenal glands each sit atop the kidneys, and produce hormones that help regulate your metabolism, immune system, blood pressure, response to stress, and other essential functions. Exactly how the adrenal gland and the liver interact is poorly understood, but we know that they do.

In most instances when speaking of adrenal problems, we are typically referring to the endocrine functions of the adrenal gland, in particular steroids, such as cortisone. The most common link goes in the direction of liver disease, resulting in adrenal impairment. For example, in patients with liver disease, 33% in one study were found to have adrenal insufficiency. In those with chronic liver failure, 65% demonstrated poor adrenal gland function. Some 95% of liver transplant patients will have poorly functioning adrenal glands.

In the vast majority of cases, the adrenal impairment is minor, but at least one report described a patient with adrenal failure

who developed severe elevation in liver enzymes. Once the adrenal problem was fixed, the liver function returned to normal in
approximately 12 days. In most instances, abnormalities in liver
enzymes are minor and easily reversed to normal levels. Yet, with
severe liver failure we see a high incidence of adrenal failure,
which is correlated with the severity of the liver disorder.

There are other endocrine problems, such as diabetes and
abnormal thyroid function, that are commonly associated with
liver impairment, usually showing elevated liver enzymes. It is
known that 10 to 20% of diabetics have elevated liver enzymes,
usually of a minor degree. Again, it depends on the severity of
the diabetes. Hyperthyroidism is also associated with elevation
in certain liver enzymes. The ALP enzyme is elevated in 64% of
people with hyperthyroidism, and the ALT enzyme is elevated in
35% of these patients.

Gallbladder Disease

The gallbladder is a small pear-shaped sac located underneath the
liver. Its function is to store the bile your liver produces and pass it
along a duct that empties into the small intestine, where it helps
in the digestion of food.

"Gallbladder disease," is an umbrella term that refers to problems that affect the gallbladder. One of the most common of
these is gallstones, which are small, hard, crystalline masses often
formed from cholesterol, or other types of deposits in the bile.

Gallstones constitute one of the most common gastrointestinal disorders requiring hospitalization. Some 20 to 25 million
people in the U.S., or 10 to 15% of the population, have gallstones. The highest incidence is found in Native Americans (60 to
70%) with Hispanics with mixed Indian heritage having the sec-
ond-highest incidence. The lowest incidence is seen in Asians and

Africans (less than 5%). Approximately 10 to 15% of Caucasians have gallstones.

The major risk factors include being female, pregnancy, obesity, rapid weight loss, liver cirrhosis, hemolytic anemia, increase in blood triglycerides, metabolic syndrome, terminal ileal resection, reduced physical activity, and the use of estrogens, oral contraceptives, and certain medications (clofibrate and Ceftriaxone). Having more than one of these conditions or exposures greatly increases one's risk.

In Western countries, 75 to 80% of all gallstones are composed of cholesterol. Poor gallbladder motility is commonly linked to the risk of developing such stones. By motility, I mean the ability of the gallbladder to contract, which empties its contents into the duodenum by way of the bile duct. When the gallbladder empties poorly, it becomes distended and the bile within the gallbladder stagnates, forming cholesterol stones.

Bacteria within the gallbladder also increases the formation of stones by two major processes: one is by forming a nidus, or infected area, for the stone to grow around, and the other is by causing inflammation within the wall of the gallbladder. Magnesium reduces gallstones, mainly by reducing inflammation.

The compound curcumin, an extract of the spice turmeric, has several beneficial effects on the liver and in preventing gallstones. Most importantly, turmeric stimulates the gallbladder to contract, thus preventing stagnation of the bile. It is also a very powerful anti-inflammatory and has antibacterial properties as well.

Curcumin helps protect the liver from many inflammatory diseases. Cirrhosis and hepatocellular carcinoma (the most common type of liver cancer) are both the result of chronic liver inflammation. Curcumin also alters a number of cell-signaling processes that are critical for the growth of cancers. Other beneficial substances include silymarin, quercetin, baicalin, and hesperidin. The nano-form of these flavonoids greatly increases their effectiveness by drastically improving absorption and allowing these plant-derived compounds to enter liver cells. These can be purchased from the One Planet Nutrition company (www.oneplanetnutrition.com).

Obesity and Liver Disease

Obesity, especially visceral obesity (often called a "beer gut"), increases the risk of developing a number of diseases, such as diabetes, neurodegenerative diseases, heart attacks, heart failure, atherosclerosis, strokes, and certain cancers. Obesity is also associated with liver disorders and worsens these liver diseases, mostly by causing them to progress rapidly and extensively.

Studies have shown that for every 1% increase in visceral fat (fat around your intestines) there is a doubling of fats deposited within the liver. Obesity is strongly linked to developing non-alcoholic fatty liver disease (NAFLD—also covered in Chapter 13.). The reason visceral fat is a greater danger than fat under your skin (subcutaneous fat) is that when the fatty acids (triglycerides) are released from the visceral fat cells, it is released into the hepatic portal system of veins, which carries the fat directly to the liver.

One answer to the mystery as to why visceral fat is deadlier than subcutaneous fat is that the former fat is infiltrated with numerous immune cells called *macrophages*. These are highly inflammatory cells and raise inflammation throughout the body, including the liver. That means that the fat deposited within the liver is causing inflammation of the liver, which is compounded by the general body inflammation caused by the visceral fat itself.

One study demonstrated that compared to normal controls, obese people demonstrated a 4.6-fold increase in fatty livers.

Another study found that 76% of obese people who never drank had fatty livers, whereas only 10 to 15% of normal-weight individuals had fatty livers.

The incidence of fatty liver disease varies significantly with ethnicity, with a 45% incidence in Hispanics, 33% in whites, and 24% in blacks. The incidence was almost twice as high in males as females (42% vs. 24%, respectively).

Many obese individuals can have fatty liver disease without any outward sign they are having problems. Yet, as the disease progresses and the liver becomes more damaged, problems begin to arise.

Insulin resistance, the impaired cellular response to insulin, may be a major link between having fatty liver disease (NAFLD) and obesity. Insulin resistance is very common with obesity. You will recall that insulin resistance is associated with high levels of free radical generation and lipid peroxidation, which damages numerous liver structures and magnifies liver inflammation.

Unfortunately, most doctors screen patients for liver problems by getting liver enzyme tests, such as ALT (alanine aminotransferase). Studies have shown that patients with well-defined fatty liver disease can have perfectly normal liver enzymes. Depending on tests demonstrating elevated liver enzymes is not a good way to diagnose fatty liver problems. Ultrasonography, a non-invasive test that uses soundwaves, is almost 4 times more effective at assessing the presence of fatty liver disease.

The problem with a delayed diagnosis is that benign fatty liver disease can rapidly progress to inflammatory liver disease (NASH or nonalcoholic steatohepatitis), which appreciably raises the risk of developing advanced cirrhosis or even liver cancer. Factors that strongly indicate a high risk of advancing toward liver fibrosis include obesity combined with insulin resistance and high triglyceride blood levels. Of these, the strongest predictor was obesity. Interestingly, curcumin (Nano-Curcumin) power-fully reduces the risk of liver fibrosis.

To appreciate just how dangerous obesity really is, one study found that obesity with hidden early cirrhosis was equal to hav-ing hepatitis C in terms of the risk of developing cirrhosis and hepatocellular carcinoma (liver cancer).

If all this is not frightening enough, it has been shown that a combination of diabetes, obesity, and fatty liver disease (NAFLD) was associated with poor survival and is a leading cause of death. People who are not obese and have NAFLD are not at a signifi-cantly increased risk of death, but the obese person with NAFLD is at a very high risk of dying. Keep in mind that obesity, especially abdominal obesity, causes chronic high levels of inflammation throughout the body, including in the brain, and it causes addi-tional inflammation within the liver. Because obesity is linked to insulin resistance, the risk becomes even higher. Losing the excess fat puts one back into a much lower-risk category.

CHAPTER 11

Diabetes and Your Liver

Diabetes, known also as diabetes mellitus, is the seventh most common cause of death in our nation, and also a major contributor to many top serious disorders, including heart disease, nerve damage, kidney disease, blindness, and amputations. In addition, diabetes is also linked to several neurodegenerative disorders, including Alzheimer's disease. Diabetes affects the body's ability to use glucose (sugar), and because all of the body's tissues depend on this nutrient, diabetes can result in extensive damage in every tissue and organ in the body.

The fact that this disease is also a major cause of liver disease is often completely overlooked by many physicians, and more so by the public. Indeed, diabetes is linked to several liver disorders, including fatty liver disease (NAFLD and NASH), liver fibrosis, cirrhosis, liver cancer, and acute liver failure, and is also linked to hepatitis C. Pre-diabetes, which is even more prevalent, is increasing in the world at an alarming rate, especially in the U.S. Insulin resistance and the metabolic syndrome (a cluster of conditions occurring together that increase heart disease risk) are also important links to diabetes mellitus. There is a very strong connection among metabolic syndrome, insulin resistance, and fatty liver diseases, as noted in previous chapters.

There are two basic types of diabetes: insulin dependent or type 1 diabetes, known also as juvenile diabetes, and insulin resistant (glucose intolerance) diabetes, called type 2 diabetes. Type 2 diabetes is by far the most common type and is increasing at a very high rate in the U.S.

A juvenile form of diabetes can develop in small children and is related to early life exposure to cow's milk in children with a particular genetic defect. It can also occur as a result of viral infections and as a response to vaccinations. Dr. Bart Classen, who I know personally, found in his research that there is a strong connection between certain vaccines during childhood and type 1 diabetes. Other studies have shown a significant connection between a low vitamin D_3 level and the incidence of type 1 diabetes. Dark-skinned people have the highest incidence of type 2 diabetes, and also the lowest levels of vitamin D_3.

The strongest connections to type 2 diabetes include obesity, consuming fructose, and one's total consumption of sugars. Research also links inflammation, which is universal with obesity and insulin resistance. Because of the widespread use of high-fructose corn syrup, we are now seeing a frightening increase in both obesity and type 2 diabetes. This epidemic of obesity, metabolic syndrome, and type 2 diabetes has now spread to our youth in alarming numbers. Fatty liver disease (NAFLD) is now epidemic in the world, especially in the U.S., and is directly related to the use of fructose and sucrose (table sugar), the latter of which contains both fructose and glucose.

Given these facts, it's obvious that preventing diabetes, and those lifestyle habits that lead to diabetes, is keenly important if you want to safeguard your liver's health. Controlling insulin sensitivity is also important in treating established liver diseases.

How Common Is Diabetes?

In the U.S., diabetes has grown to epidemic proportions, with the number of diagnosed cases having tripled since 1980. The American Diabetes Association now estimates there are as many as 29 million Americans living with type 2 diabetes—that's approximately 8% of the population. As bad as these figures sound, it is estimated that 86 million (more than one in three people) have pre-diabetes—that is, early changes that, more often than not, go undetected until serious events happen.

Worldwide, approximately 1 in 10 adults have type 2 diabetes. The number of people with this disorder has more than doubled, from 153 million in 1980, to 347 million in 2008. Estimates of global pre-diabetes have not been available, but at present trends, this silent disorder could affect billions of people.

What Is the Liver's Role?

Diabetes is a metabolic disorder that interferes with the body's ability to metabolize blood glucose (sugar). Interference with glucose metabolism, while basically related to impaired entry of glucose into cells, ultimately involves several harmful effects on cells, tissue, and organs, which can result in a number of serious disorders.

Sugar is important and necessary for your body to function, but in excess, it acts as a poison, especially to the brain. Neuroscientists call the toxicity of excess sugar in the brain glucotoxicity. We get most of the sugar from the food we eat, but it is also the job of both the liver and kidneys to produce it naturally.

The liver plays an extremely important role by both manufacturing and storing glucose, fuel for our bodies. The liver has a storage form of sugar called *glycogen*. It can also convert fats and proteins into sugars when these glycogen stores are depleted. Glucose's main advantage is that it can instantly supply energy to the cells, whereas the release from glycogen stores, and especially the conversion from fats and proteins, occurs rather slowly.

Normally, the liver releases its glucose in small amounts, to prevent a strain on insulin release from the pancreas. When glucose levels are very high in the blood, the insulin-producing cells in the pancreas (called the *islets of Langerhans*) must produce very high levels of insulin to bring the sugar down to normal levels. This can, over time, cause such stress on these insulin producing cells as to cause them to die. When that happens, the type 2 diabetes converts to type 1 diabetes—that is, insulin dependent, which means the person needs to be given insulin injections on a regular basis.

The fact that the liver impacts the pancreas can be seen in the connection between fatty liver disease and diabetes, as discussed earlier. Some studies have found that slim people who aren't considered ordinarily to be at risk for diabetes, can have fatty livers. Yet, in most cases there is a strong connection between obesity and having a fatty liver.

Type 2 Diabetes: The Most Common Form of Diabetes

Type 2 diabetes is the most common form of the disease, accounting for 90 to 95% of cases.

Marked by elevated levels of blood sugar and insulin, type 2 diabetes is characterized by normal insulin-producing capacity from the pancreas. The disease develops when there is a malfunction in insulin receptors on the surface of cells. Insulin interacts with these insulin receptors on the cell surface to allow glucose to enter the cell. With type 2 diabetes having defective insulin receptors, the cells are unable to take up the sugar from the blood, and, as a result, levels of both insulin and glucose in the blood become chronically elevated. This impairment is also described as insulin resistance because the cells are literally resistant to the normal functioning of insulin.

The incidence of diabetes is growing at unprecedented levels, as the incidence of obesity, lack of physical activity, and a poor diet become more prevalent.

High levels of insulin, which can occur with insulin resistance, can also cause damage itself, mainly in the form of inflammation. Damage to blood vessels (atherosclerosis), the retinas, brain damage, and damage to other organs, especially the kidneys and heart, are all caused by the chronic inflammation triggered by insulin resistance. Insulin also stimulates the accumulation of fats in fat cells, especially in the most dangerous fat—visceral fat.

Visceral fat is the fat within your abdomen, mainly surrounding your intestines and internal organs. This type of fat is most strongly associated with insulin resistance and inflammation. We most often associate visceral fat with the "pot belly" appearance, but thin people or people of normal size can have excess visceral fat. Excess visceral fat is also associated with sleep apnea, and reduction of the fat, or even its surgical removal, has been shown to cure sleep apnea in a number of cases.

Symptoms of Type 2 Diabetes

- Being hungry after eating
- Feeling tired frequently
- Being very thirsty
- Urinating often
- Losing weight without reason
- Numbness in the hands or feet

- Blurry vision
- Sores that heal very slowly

Symptoms of type 2 diabetes can appear very gradually. Which is why I refer to it in the early stages as "silent diabetes" (pre-diabetes).

Researchers once believed that the average time between the onset of diabetes and its diagnosis was 7 to 10 years, but new research finds that early signs of this disorder may occur even earlier than that. This means that type 2 diabetes has a tremendous head start in damaging your body, including your liver.

What Is Insulin Resistance?

Early stage insulin resistance, known also as pre-diabetes, is a condition that is a silent precursor to diabetes. Basically, as symptoms begin to appear, we have a warning sign that tells you that, if you don't change your lifestyle, and primarily lose weight and change your diet, you are at very high risk of developing diabetes. The good news is that you can reverse insulin resistance with weight loss, several natural flavonoid products, and a change in one's diet.

Newer studies are showing that natural compounds isolated from specific plants, such as berberine, can correct insulin resistance and prevent the damage caused by this disorder.

What Causes Diabetes?

Obesity is the chief link to type 2 diabetes.

If you are overweight, the likelihood you will become diabetic soars. While this is especially true if diabetes runs in your family, obesity trumps even genetics, so if you gain weight in middle age, you increase your risk, even if you have no relatives with the disease. This is true even if you gain only a small amount of weight in mid-life, although the more weight you gain, the higher your risk. Again, the most important type of fat gain is visceral fat, not the fat under your skin (subcutaneous fat).

Several plant flavonoids can selectively reduce visceral fat, as mentioned previously, and are therefore more likely to correct your diabetes and even metabolic syndrome.

How Is Diabetes Treated?

In people with diabetes, controlling blood sugar through diet, oral medications, or insulin is the main treatment. Regular screening for complications is also required.

Type 2 diabetes had been considered an incurable disease, but we now know that, with regular exercise, a healthy diet, the use of plant flavonoids and other special natural compounds, and weight loss, this disorder can be prevented, and even reversed.

However, many doctors have not yet gotten that message, and are not trained to help patients effectively change their lifestyle.

Type 2 Diabetes *Is* Reversible!

It's generally believed, even by much of the medical profession, that, once you develop type 2 diabetes, you're stuck with it for life. But thanks to new research, we now have scientific proof that this isn't true.

In a landmark study, recently published in *Lancet*, UK investigators randomly assigned nearly 300 people who had been diagnosed with type 2 diabetes to one of two groups: a weight management program, or one in which they continued with their usual treatments and diets.

After a year, most of the people in the antidiabetic diet group lost about 22 pounds, compared to 2 pounds in the control group. However, and most importantly, 46% of the people in the diet group reversed their diabetes, meaning they went into remission, compared to just 4% in the control group.

In 2002, the Diabetes Prevention Program study showed that diet and exercise alone could prevent people with pre-diabetes from progressing to full-blown diabetes, in some cases better than with medications designed to control blood glucose. But this study goes further, and demonstrates that reversal is possible, even with people who have been diagnosed with the full-blown disorder.

The study included people who had been living with the diagnosis for 6 years or less. The investigators admitted they had no evidence if one would get the same results with people having diabetes longer.

A growing number of studies and personal experience demonstrates that the proper use of special nutritional compounds can safely and effectively correct most cases of type 2 diabetes, and most importantly, reduce the complications associated with long-term diabetes. Diabetics suffer from a number of serious complications, which include:

- Blindness
- Cataracts
- Impotence in men
- Kidney failure
- Rapid atherosclerosis (amputation of limbs)
- Heart failure
- Strokes
- Liver failure

- Dysbiosis (an imbalance in the gut bacteria)
- Neurodegenerative diseases
- Peripheral neuropathy
- Muscle loss
- Pulmonary disorders
- Frequent infections (immune suppression)
- Increased cancer rates

Tips on Weight Loss

As you've seen, one of the keys in reversing diabetes is weight loss. Here are some tips:

Fruits and Vegetables: Moderation Is the Rule

Fruits contain varying amounts of sugars and should only be eaten in limited amounts. Some people gain weight with any sugar exposure. They should avoid whole fruits, but can use fruit extracts that have removed the sugar. Vegetables contain fewer sugars and moderate amounts of complex carbohydrates, which are better tolerated. The importance of vegetables is that they contain a number of flavonoid compounds that reduce free radical damage and lipid peroxidation, a major problem seen with diabetes. Complex carbohydrates are slowly converted into glucose in the body, allowing time for metabolism to prevent fat gain, but only if eaten in moderation.

Eat Protein in Moderation

Animal protein plays an important role in good health for a number of reasons. Most of your proteins should come from organically fed animals. Newer studies have shown that the caution being spread by many health agencies about the dangers of meat consumption is not accurate and that organically raised meats contain healthy oils and flavonoids (naturally occurring compounds in fruits and vegetables) needed for good health, as well as balanced proteins. Non-organically raised meats contain high levels of pesticides, herbicides, fungicides, and industrial chemicals (concentrated in the fats) that can worsen the damage caused by diabetes. Beef should not be eaten cooked rare because most cattle populations contain carcinogenic and neurotropic viruses in the tissues. In some herds, researchers found carcinogenic viruses in 80% of the animals examined. Heat will kill these viruses, but they survive in rare-cooked meats. Studies have shown that even handlers of raw meats in slaughterhouses have a significantly higher incidence of hemopoietic malignancies (leukemia, lymphoma, and multiple myeloma).

Fiber: The Good and Bad

Foods that are high in fiber, including many vegetables and fruits (with the skins on if organic), benefit you in two ways: First, they'll fill you up and help reduce hunger, and they reduce colon cancer incidence. Soluble fiber is particularly beneficial. Great sources of soluble fiber include strawberries, oat bran, citrus fruits, inulin, and chicory. Soluble fiber is used by the colon bacteria as a food. Studies have shown that only vegetable fiber prevents cancer, not grain fiber.

Here are other sources of fiber:

- **Legumes.** Beans, peas, and nuts are some of the best sources of soluble fiber you can find. Beans are rich in protein and fill you up. Beans are a fairly good source of some antioxidants. It is important that all beans be cooked thoroughly because they have high levels of lectins, which can harm your health. Some beans, such as black beans, are also high in glutamate, an excitotoxin. Excitotoxins stimulate the growth of cancers and can damage the liver, especially a liver that is already damaged.

- **Brussels sprouts and broccoli.** Vegetables are good sources of soluble fiber, and both Brussels sprouts and broccoli are at the top of the list. (Sweet potatoes and asparagus are also good.) As with the beans, they need to be cooked well, because they are also high in lectins. They should be cooked either by steaming or cooking in water. Both contain a number of antioxidant flavonoids, have powerful anticancer properties, protect the cardiovascular system, and are a brain protectant.

- **Blueberries and other berries.** Many different kinds of berries—including blackberries, strawberries, and raspberries—offer a wide array of health benefits. All three have powerful anticancer effectiveness, especially blackberries and raspberries. All three help keep the heart's blood vessels healthy by strengthening the vessels and reducing free radical and lipid peroxidation within the walls of these vessels—the cause of atherosclerosis. Blueberries and strawberries have been shown to be foods that not only prevent brain aging but can also reverse some of the damage seen with aging of the brain. These two berries also contain a compound (fisetin in strawberries and pterostilbene in blueberries) that reverses the aging process significantly (called a *senolytics*). Citrus fruits, such as oranges, also rank high on the soluble fiber list, but should be eaten only in limited amounts because of their sugar content. Because of the high sugar content of blueberries, it may be preferable to take blueberry extract capsules that concentrate the most effective components of the blueberry without the sugar. Blueberries are also very high in pterostilbene, which is converted in the body into resveratrol. The advantage of pterostilbene is that it is far better absorbed than resveratrol. This compound is a major liver protector.

Use Olive Oil

You hear a lot these days about substituting so-called healthy fats for saturated or trans fats such as butter or margarine. Margarine is made from a polyunsaturated omega-6 oil (usually corn oil) that is highly oxidized and therefore a major cause of free radical and lipid peroxidation damage in tissues such as the liver. An excess of omega-6 oils is very harmful, because they are pro-inflammatory and stimulate cancer growth and spread. Butter is preferable. But, of all the "good fats" out there, the one I really recommend is high-quality, cold-pressed, extra virgin olive oil, which has been found to prevent blood from excessive clotting, reduces the risk of cancer, protects the brain, and helps normalize blood glucose levels. It can be used for cooking but not at high heat. It is best to sprinkle turmeric over the oil and mix well. This extract adds antioxidant and anticancer benefits to the oil. It also adds considerably to the taste.

Avoid All Dairy Products

Dairy products are associated with a number of health problems, including an increased incidence of heart attacks and strokes. In fact, studies have shown that low-fat milk has a higher associated risk of heart attacks than whole milk. Cow's milk is also strongly associated with juvenile diabetes and is on the list of foods commonly associated with allergies. Milk, being high in calcium and glutamate, stimulates the growth of cancers.

Avoid Breads, Biscuits, and All Products
Made with Wheat, Barley, and Rye

Grains are major sources of gluten, which is associated with a number of disorders, including brain disorders such as autism, ADHD, and neurodegeneration. The best way to lose fat weight is to avoid all grains, especially breads and pasta. Pasta is very high in glutamate, a cancer promoter, and causes damage to the liver (especially if combined with aspartame). Modern breads and wheat products contain added gluten, and many processed foods contain carrageenan, which is a major inflammatory compound and cancer promoter. Recent studies have shown that when gluten is consumed in high concentrations, it can be harmful to everyone, not just people with so-called gluten intolerance.

If You Must Snack, Snack Wisely

Snacking is the great American pastime, but you need to choose your snacks wisely and eat them in small portions. One bad effect of snacking is that it becomes a habit. It also denies the intestines a chance to rest, which is important for their repair. If one must snack, nuts may be a better choice. Walnuts contain high levels of ellagic acid, which protects the blood vessels and has powerful anticancer effects. The downside is that all nuts have rather high levels of glutamate, an excitotoxin. It is best to eat these nuts in small amounts. Allergies to nuts are very common. Dark chocolate is another snack that has been found to have healthy benefits for the heart and brain. A couple of small squares make a special treat. People with migraine headaches, however, should avoid chocolate and most nuts. The glutamate in nuts can trigger serious migraine attacks.

Avoid Fruit Juices and Sweetened Drinks

Fruit juices contain high levels of sugars, which as a liquid are rapidly absorbed and raise blood sugar to higher levels. Distilled or filtered water (they must also remove fluoride) is preferred. Tea is also a great beverage, but black tea contains high levels of aluminum and fluoride (fluoroaluminum), which is associated with damage to all cells and especially the brain. White tea is the healthiest tea, with green tea a second best. One can use monk fruit as a sweetener, as it has no metabolic activity. White and green teas contain compounds called *catechins* (EGCG is the most abundant and powerful), which have numerous health benefits. Catechins bind iron, thus preventing iron excess. Tea compounds have significant anticancer effects.

Should You Be Tested for Diabetes?

According to recent studies, one in four Americans have diabetes but don't know it. An even higher percentage have pre-diabetes, the earliest stages of diabetes. Because diabetes generally causes no symptoms for years after its onset, it has a head start on damaging your body while you don't even realize it. This is why diabetes screening is so important. The simplest way to screen for diabetes in people without symptoms is with a urinalysis.

A glucose number at or slightly below 100 is normal. Any glucose number over 100 is cause for suspicion and should be addressed through weight loss and lifestyle changes. If your blood sugar is slightly above this level, it is best to have it repeated in a few weeks to a month to see if it is progressively rising.

You should be tested for diabetes if you are over the age of 45 and you have one or more of the following risk factors:

- A history of cardiovascular disease

- Are inactive
- Are overweight or obese
- Have a parent, brother, or sister with diabetes
- Have a family background that is African American, Alaska Native, American Indian, Asian American, Hispanic/Latino, or Pacific Islander
- Gave birth to a baby weighing more than 9 pounds or have been diagnosed with gestational diabetes, which is a temporary form of diabetes that occurs during pregnancy
- Have high blood pressure
- Have a triglyceride level above 250 mg/dL
- Have an elevated hs-CRP level
- Have polycystic ovary syndrome, also called PCOS
- Have other conditions associated with insulin resistance, such as a condition called *acanthosis nigricans*, characterized by a dark, velvety rash around the neck or armpits

Natural Supplements to Control Blood Sugar

A number of natural compounds have been found to reduce the effects of both type 2 (insulin resistant) diabetes and type 1 (insulin dependent) diabetes. Unlike the pharmaceuticals used to treat diabetes, many of these natural compounds also reduce inflammation as well as blood sugar. They also have the advantage of being much safer and have far fewer side effects, most of which are minor.

In addition, the compounds reduce free radical and lipid peroxidation damage, which are the most harmful mechanisms associated with diabetes. When insulin function is impaired, cells produce massive numbers of free radicals and lipid peroxidation products, which also dramatically increase inflammation. This combination of oxidative stress and inflammation produces most of the tissue and organ damage seen with both types of diabetes.

Taking drugs to improve insulin secretion, or taking insulin itself, can improve a diabetic's insulin function. The problem is that it's difficult to balance the dose of medications with one's diet. The medications can also have serious side effects. Complications associated with diabetes drugs can arise from either overdoing the dose or not taking a large enough dose.

Uncorrected diabetes can lead to a continuous production of destructive free radicals and lipid peroxidation products, which produce what are referred to as advanced glycation end products (AGEs). These damage proteins, lipids, and carbohydrates, and this interferes with the cell's ability to function. We see this as liver damage, blindness, impotence, aggressive atherosclerosis, cardio-vascular disease, kidney failure, and impaired brain function.

The beauty of using natural compounds is that they not only improve insulin function; they are also powerful antioxidants, reduce AGEs, and reduce inflammation. The most effective include:

- Nano-Berberine
- R-lipoic acid
- Nano-Quercetin
- Nano-Curcumin
- Nano-Ginger extract
- Nano-Boswellia

Nano-Berberine and Nano-Boswellia

Among these, Nano-Boswellia is especially interesting because it has been shown in multiple studies to prevent and improve both type 1 and type 2 diabetes. These studies demonstrated that boswellia prevents the autoimmune destruction of the pancre-atic insulin-producing cells (the islets of Langerhans), which cause type 1 (insulin dependent) diabetes. Boswellia does this by preventing immune lymphocyte cells from invading the insulin-producing cells, and by lowering inflammatory cytokine levels in the blood.

Another interesting compound is berberine (Nano-Berberine), which lowers blood glucose in diabetics and greatly improves lipid profiles by lowering total cholesterol and LDL cholesterol levels. Berberine, in higher doses, has been shown to completely correct type 2 diabetes in a number of people and improve blood sugar control in type 1 diabetes.

In one study, using berberine, involving patients with type 2 diabetes, researchers found a significant improvement in blood sugar and glycated hemoglobin (HbA1c) levels, along with much lower total cholesterol and LDL cholesterol levels. HbA1c is a way doctors measure long-term blood sugar control, and is a much more accurate measure than a single blood sugar test. Another study involving 116 patients with type 2 diabetes found a significant correction of blood glucose, HbA1c, and abnormal blood lipids, as well as weight loss.

A compounding pharmacist I know reported complete blood sugar control among a large number of diabetic patients—including some who were insulin-dependent—who took Nano-Berberine. He notes that higher doses worked best, as high as 500 mg three times a day with meals. Nano-Berberine is absorbed better than conventional berberine (from One Planet Nutrition, Inc.—www.oneplanetnutrition.com). A dose of 250 mg with each daily meal may be sufficient. Higher doses can be taken as needed.

Nano-Boswellia can be taken in a dose of 250 mg to 500 mg three times a day with meals.

R-Lipoic Acid

R-lipoic acid is a natural substance found in every cell in the body. It is one of the cell's most important, powerful, and versatile antioxidants. As an antioxidant, it is unusual in that it removes free radicals even when it is oxidized, which makes it the centerpiece of all antioxidant regeneration. It also powerfully lowers elevated blood sugar, even in cases of insulin-dependent (type 1) diabetes.

The R-lipoic acid form of the product is much more powerful as an antioxidant and reducer of blood sugar than is the older version called *alpha-lipoic acid*. It is very safe and has few side effects. It can cause hypoglycemia in people with reactive hypoglycemia, especially if taken on an empty stomach.

What to do. For type 1 diabetes, the dose is 600 to 800 mg of R-lipoic acid with each meal. For type 2 diabetes, the dose would be 300 to 600 mg taken with each meal. It can be mixed with the other blood sugar–lowering flavonoids, but the doses may have to be adjusted. One should follow blood sugar measurement to adjust the dose. It should be mixed with antidiabetic medications only under the guidance of one's doctor. In many cases of type 2 diabetes, a person can stop taking such medications. Blood sugars must be carefully monitored.

Nano-Quercetin

Like curcumin, quercetin is a powerful antioxidant, anti-inflammatory, antidiabetic, and anti-infection compound. It is found in many fruits and vegetables, being especially high in teas, onions, and garlic. Quercetin can lower blood sugar effectively when it is elevated. The main problem is it is poorly absorbed from the stomach and intestines. Nano-Quercetin is far better absorbed and effective.

What to do. Nano-Quercetin can be taken with the other antidiabetic compounds listed earlier, but one should carefully monitor his or her blood sugar to adjust the doses. It should be taken with food no more than 20 minutes before eating. The usual dose is one 250 mg capsule taken three times a day with meals. Higher doses can be used as needed.

Magnesium Citrate/Malate

Magnesium is one of the essential minerals in the body and is involved in the operation of over 200 enzyme reactions. Depletion of magnesium is very common in diabetes and greatly increases inflammation and metabolic disruptions. Magnesium depletion in the liver is very common with NASH, liver fibrosis, and cirrhosis. All states of inflammation cause a depletion of magnesium from the body, which further aggravates the inflammation.

A number of magnesium supplements are available. The least expensive is magnesium sulfate and magnesium chloride. Unfortunately, both are associated with diarrhea, mainly because these forms are poorly absorbed from the intestines. Absorption of these two forms varies widely among people.

A more absorbable form, and therefore less likely to cause diarrhea, is magnesium malate and magnesium citrate. The slow-release form, made by www.jigsawhealth.com, contains magnesium malate.

What to do. The usual dose is two slow-release tablets twice a day with a meal. Even though it is less likely to cause diarrhea, it still can. Taking the tablets with a meal reduces this risk.

Cinnamon Extract

A relative of the turmeric plant, cinnamon has been shown to significantly improve insulin function and lower elevated blood sugar. It also reduces inflammation. In my experience, it is not as beneficial as Nano-Berberine, however.

What to do. It is important to use a pure cinnamon extract and not cinnamon bark. For benefits, the dose varies widely, from 1000 to 6000 mg a day.

Nano-Curcumin

A recent study found that curcumin can not only prevent diabetes from occurring, it can also greatly improve elevated blood sugar and correct insulin resistance. In addition, it can prevent, to a large extent, the atherosclerosis buildup associated with diabetes. Curcumin is a very powerful anti-inflammatory, neutralizes dangerous free radicals and lipid peroxidation products, and protects the brain. The best form to take is Nano-Curcumin, which contains 250 mg per capsule and is a highly absorbed product. Curcumin binds iron, and if taken over a prolonged period, it can cause significant iron loss. To prevent this, vitamin C can be taken with the Nano-Curcumin, because vitamin C prevents iron binding by curcumin.

What to do. Two capsules, which together contain 500 mg, taken 30 to 45 minutes before a meal will have a maximum effect. Safety for much higher doses of curcumin has been established. Nano-Curcumin by One Planet Nutrition has the highest absorption form of curcumin.

Multivitamin/Mineral

I recommend a well-balanced multivitamin and mineral supplement. The B vitamins, when possible, should be in their most functional form. Specifically, folic acid or folate should be in the form of MTHF, short for 5-methyltetrahydrofolate; vitamin B_6 should be in the form of pyridoxal 5-phosphate; and riboflavin (vitamin B_2) should be in the form of riboflavin 5'-phosphate. These forms, which are the functional forms, are much more effective for diabetes, as diabetics have difficulty converting these basic B vitamins into their functional forms. Basic Nutrients V, made by Thorne Research, is an example of such a product.

What to do. Take a multivitamin with the recommended forms of B vitamins, per product directions. The best form of thiamine (vitamin B1) is a product called Benfotiamine. It produces higher blood levels longer than regular vitamin B1, it reduces elevated blood sugar, and is highly protective of the brain. The dose is 150 mg twice a day with a meal.

Hyperbaric Oxygen Therapy (HBOT)

HBOT has been shown to improve insulin resistance, the cause of type 2 diabetes. In addition, it can reduce the risk of complications by helping to reverse two other harmful aspects of diabetes: widespread inflammation and the destruction of small blood vessels.

CHAPTER 12

The Many Types of Viral Hepatitis

Hepatitis is an inflammation of the liver. It can be mild or it can progress to liver fibrosis, liver cirrhosis, or even to a very malignant form of liver cancer called a *hepatocellular carcinoma*. Acute liver disease, which means it comes on suddenly, and lasts a short period, occurs in some cases, but often, especially with a hepatitis C viral infection, what is far more common are a chronic long lasting course of the disease. Asymptomatic cases of viral hepatitis are more dangerous because they can silently progress to more advanced cases of liver destruction over many years.

Viral hepatitis is a common cause of acute liver disease; a disease is considered acute if it develops quickly and lasts less than 6 months. A chronic liver disease usually comes on more subtly, often without obvious symptoms, and is longer lasting. Sometimes, an acute disease develops into a chronic ailment.

Types of Hepatitis

There are five different major types of hepatitis: A, B, C, D, and E, with types B and C most common in the U.S. There are three other types of hepatitis: F, G, and TT. In addition, there is also a type of hepatitis known as autoimmune hepatitis.

Hepatitis A, or HAV, is an infection of the liver that causes inflammation and flu-like symptoms, such as fatigue and fever. This form of hepatitis is rare in the U.S., and more common in developing countries. This form of hepatitis is spread mainly by contaminated foods, people having sex with multiple partners, and through homosexual sex. The virus mainly enters the colon from bile excretions from the liver and from there it is spread by inadequate handwashing and poor hygiene.

Unlike other forms of hepatitis, most hepatitis A cases are not associated with liver failure, and the person generally completely recovers without treatment. Occasional liver failure has been reported, usually in people with preexisting liver disorders.

Hepatitis D mainly affects people who have hepatitis B.

Hepatitis E is contracted through contaminated water (similar to hepatitis A), or can occur in people who already have a compromised immune system. Person-to-person transmission is rare, but it can also occur due to heterosexual sex with many partners and through homosexual sex.

Hepatitis F is a suspected form of hepatitis, but no virus has been identified. Hepatitis G is a relatively recently identified virus, but has not demonstrated disease transmission. It almost always occurs in conjunction with hepatitis A, B, or C. Hepatitis TT refers to a virus that has been identified, but there is currently no evidence it causes disease.

Autoimmune hepatitis is a rare form of hepatitis in which the immune system attacks your liver. Drug therapy with corticosteroids may slow down the condition's progression, but it may eventually progress to cirrhosis and liver failure, which necessitates a liver transplant.

The most common forms of hepatitis in the U.S. are B and C, although cases in A have been rising, so that type is included in more detail here as well. The U.S. has one of the lowest incidences of hepatitis B in the world.

Acute vs. Chronic Hepatitis

Acute hepatitis refers to a disease that comes on quickly with obvious symptoms, and disappears in less than 6 months. Chronic hepatitis can present slowly, without obvious symptoms, and lingers longer, for months or years. Acute hepatitis can also progress into the chronic form.

Hepatitis A

Hepatitis is very contagious, usually quite mild, and is rare in the U.S. It is most commonly contracted by eating food prepared by someone with the disease who did not wash their hands properly. Transmission by eating undercooked food, especially shellfish, has also been reported. Uncooked foods are a major source in endemic areas, such as salads, cold sandwiches, and some pastries. It is also spread through objects handled by an infected person (fomites). Infected children, who mainly remain asymptomatic, commonly spread the infection. In many cases, the source is an asymptomatic infected family member, usually a child under age five.

The disease is more common in developing countries. In 2015, there were only 1390 reported cases of hepatitis A in the U.S.

However, since the current outbreaks were first identified in late 2016, more than 37,000 cases have been reported, chiefly among groups most at risk. Severe complications, high rates of hospitalization, and more than 340 deaths have occurred nation-wide as a result of these outbreaks, according to the CDC.

People who travel to countries that have hepatitis A are also at risk, as well as people who anticipate close personal contact with an international adoptee.

People with chronic liver disease, including hepatitis B and hepatitis C, and people with HIV, are at increased risk.

Hepatitis A, as stated, is mainly spread through contaminated food. This contamination of food with the hepatitis A virus can happen at any point: growing, harvesting, processing, handling, and even after incomplete cooking. Contamination of food and water happens more often in countries where hepatitis A is common. Although uncommon, food-borne outbreaks have occurred in the U.S. from people eating contaminated fresh and frozen imported food products.

Hepatitis A also frequently appears in these at-risk groups:

- International travelers
- Gay and bisexual men
- People who use or inject drugs (all those who use illegal drugs)
- People with an occupational risk for exposure
- People who anticipate close personal contact with an international adoptee
- People experiencing homelessness
- People with chronic liver disease, including hepatitis B and hepatitis C
- People with HIV
- Pregnant women at risk for hepatitis A or at risk for severe outcomes from hepatitis A infections

The incubation period varies from 14 to 45 days, with a median of 28 days. The highest concentration of viruses, which are secreted primarily from bile, occurs 1 to 2 weeks before clinical symptoms occur. The number of viruses secreted decrease precipitously once clinical symptoms occur. The virus itself produces little or no damage; most of the liver injury is caused by a person's own immune system when it reacts to the virus.

While most cases are mild or asymptomatic, in rare instances fulminate hepatitis with rapid liver failure can occur. Chronic infections do not occur with this virus, but relapses can occur. Adults are more likely to develop symptoms than children, usually involving fatigue, nausea and/or vomiting, loss of appetite, a jaundice-like appearance, or dark urine.

Infections are best prevented by improving personal hygiene and sanitation. Food handlers should all wear gloves and practice sanitary handwashing after going to the bathroom.

Hepatitis B

Like hepatitis A, hepatitis B was once rare in the U.S., but is now on the increase in certain groups, such as IV drug users, those getting tattoos or piercings, practicing homosexuals, and those having many heterosexual partners, especially individuals having sex with IV drug users. Prisons also have a high incidence of hepatitis B. Outside of these high-risk groups it remains rare in the U.S.

Unlike hepatitis A, in a relatively small number of cases, hepatitis B can result in a serious liver disease. Approximately 95% of cases of hepatitis B will resolve without any specific treatment. Of the remaining 5%, some of these cases may reoccur without significant liver damage, or in 0.1 to 2% of cases, it can become a chronic infection. Chronic infections have a higher risk of progressing to liver fibrosis, cirrhosis, and of significantly increasing the risk of developing liver cancer (hepatocellular carcinoma). Cancer related to chronic hepatitis B is not a direct effect of the virus but a secondary to long-term inflammation associated with the infection.

As with the hepatitis A virus, most of the damage to the liver is not caused by the virus itself, but rather by the person's immune reaction to the virus. In addition, people with preexisting liver disorders, such as NAFLD and NASH, those with a poor nutritional status, the frail elderly, regular aspartame users, and those having regular exposure to alcohol, are much more likely to suffer from progressive liver destruction associated with chronic hepatitis B infections. Most adults fully recover from the infection without any treatment. Lifelong immunity is characteristic with recovery from natural infections, but not from vaccinations. Hepatitis B vaccinations have a very high complication rate, with a significant number of people suffering serious complications. The practice of vaccinating all newborn babies with this vaccine was a disaster. The same has been true for adults. One study, clearly demonstrated that the incidence of multiple sclerosis was drastically increased in those that had been vaccinated and could appear years after the vaccine has been taken. In addition, the vaccine protection was shown to be gone after 5 to 10 years, long before the person would ever come in contact with the virus.

The rate of hepatitis B had been declining, but in 2015 the acute hepatitis B infection rate in the U.S. increased by 20.7%, rising for the first time since 2006. The sharpest increases in new hepatitis B cases are occurring largely in states that have been impacted the most by the opioid epidemic, because the virus can spread through shared needles. Still, hepatitis B remains more common in the developing world. Each year, about 3000

Americans die from hepatitis B, compared to more than 600,000 worldwide.

The risk for chronic infection is related to age at infection: about 90% of infants with hepatitis B go on to develop a chronic infection, whereas only 2 to 5% of people who get hepatitis B as adults become chronically infected.

The virus can be transmitted through bodily fluids, such as blood, semen, and vaginal fluids, but is not spread through food or casual contact.

Symptoms of Hepatitis B

Children under the age of five, and about one-third of older children and adults, do not have symptoms, but over a period of years, or decades, they have a small risk of developing chronic liver disease and liver failure, which can lead to disability or even death. Generally, symptoms appear between 6 weeks and 6 months after exposure to the virus, most often after about 3 months, and may include:

- Fatigue
- Loss of appetite
- Fever
- Stomach pain
- Dark urine
- Nausea
- Vomiting
- Joint pain
- Bowel movements that are clay-colored
- Jaundice (yellow skin or eyes)

Conventional Treatments

While antiviral medications are used for acute hepatitis B infections, they do not prevent recurrences, and most are associated with many complications, some serious. Once diagnosed, however, an individual should take precautions not to spread the disease.

For chronic infections, medications are not necessarily recommended because of side effects. However, the health of the liver should be monitored, alcohol should be avoided, and any prescription or over-the-counter drugs that may harm the liver should be avoided, such as acetaminophen. Liver damaging artificial sweeteners, such as aspartame, sucralose (Splenda), acesulfame, and saccharine should also be avoided. Alcohol in all forms should be avoided.

Hepatitis C

Hepatitis C was not identified until 1989. Prior to that, it was referred to as Non-A, Non-B hepatitis. There are several genotypes and a number of subtypes of the virus, each having a different viral behavior, complication rate, geographic distribution, and cure rate.

The virus is usually spread through blood, and less often through fluids exchanged during sex, but not through kissing, hugging, shaking hands, coughing, sneezing, food, or water. Its incidence is rising in the U.S. The sharing of needles by drug addicts is a major source of the disease. Blood transfusions are another source, although in the U.S., donated blood is screened for the virus and a few other pathogens.

A review from 2013 through 2016 estimated that there are over 2 million people in the U.S. infected with this virus, making it the most common blood-borne infection in the country.

Chronic liver damage associated with this virus accounts for the greatest number of liver transplants. The incidence of hepatitis C is half that of hepatitis B, but has a much higher incidence of liver cirrhosis, making it a more dangerous disease. Individuals infected with the HIV virus develop liver cirrhosis much sooner than otherwise healthy people.

Western countries account for only a small portion of the global cases, with 50% of hepatitis C cases occurring in five countries—China, Pakistan, India, Egypt, and Russia. In general, infections contracted by drug users are among younger individuals, and those getting the infection from medical contamination (iatrogenic) are older.

Like hepatitis B, hepatitis C is also a viral infection that causes liver inflammation and can, in a number of cases, lead to serious liver damage, mainly because in most cases there are few if any symptoms, thus allowing progressive liver destruction to occur unknown to the person. The virus can also present as an acute or chronic infection, and lead to the same dangerous conditions as hepatitis B does, only causing a higher incidence of chronic liver damage. The incidence of this virus in the U.S. has been rising. There is no vaccine for hepatitis C.

Hepatitis C is a big problem for Baby Boomers. Americans born between 1945 and 1964 are five times more likely to develop the infection, for reasons that are not completely understood. The symptoms of hepatitis C can be vague, meaning that people in a high-risk category should be tested even though they have no symptoms. This is especially important because, unlike a minor number of hepatitis B cases, which are manageable but not curable, hepatitis C is mostly curable.

Especially if left untreated, chronic hepatitis C can result in scarring (fibrosis) that can eventually lead to cirrhosis. If not halted or reversed, cirrhosis leads to liver failure and rapid death.

Hepatitis C is also dangerous because it can cause complications resulting in other disorders. These potential complications include:

- Cryoglobulinemia, a condition that causes abnormal proteins to clump together in the blood
- Hepatic fibrosis and eventual cirrhosis
- Non-Hodgkin's lymphoma
- Insulin resistance and eventual diabetes
- Chronic fatigue
- Kidney disease
- Skin conditions
- Vasculitis (inflammation of the blood vessels)

As with other causes of liver cirrhosis, chronic hepatitis C is associated with a higher incidence of hepatocellular carcinoma, a deadly form of liver cancer. Globally, there were 895,000 deaths from this cancer in 1990, which increased to 1,454,000 cancer deaths in 2013. Infection by this virus without accompanying liver cirrhosis is rarely associated with hepatocellular carcinoma. Over a 20- to 30-year span, 75 to 85% of those with asymptomatic infections will develop liver cirrhosis.

Most people who are infected have no symptoms, but in rare acute cases, they may experience fatigue, loss of appetite, fever, stomach pain, dark urine, nausea, vomiting, joint pain, bowel movements that are clay-colored, or jaundice (yellow skin or eyes). This virus, in the long run, is more serious than the hepatitis B virus.

With the appearance of liver cirrhosis, one may experience a buildup of fluid in the abdomen (called *ascites*), develop upper GI (gastrointestinal) bleeding, experience kidney damage or failure, and suddenly develop lethargy, stupor, have difficulty thinking, and eventually slip into a coma—all of which is part of a condition called *hepatic encephalopathy*. Kidney failure is 10 times more common with chronic infections than is seen in the healthy population. Liver cirrhosis is more commonly seen in people who abuse alcohol, are older, have a co-infection with hepatitis B virus or HIV virus, or have other infections.

It is estimated that there are approximately 15 million cases of cirrhosis worldwide, with one million cases leading to a complete loss of liver function, requiring either liver transplantation or leading to death.

Diagnostic Testing

Most diagnoses are made using serum or a plasma anti-HCV test, which is a highly specific test. A rapid finger prick test is also available for screening. Conversion from a negative test to a positive test is usually diagnostic. The anti-HCV test can remain positive years after one is cured. For determining an active infection, one may require HCV RNA testing or real-time PCR testing. The PCR test can only diagnose infection in symptomatic individuals and can have a high degree of inaccuracy if not done properly.

The elevation of liver enzymes—ALT and AST—is suspicious but not diagnostic, as many conditions can cause this. Many infected people can have no liver enzyme elevation. Testing cases of more severe liver damage is critical in cases of known infection, specifically when looking for signs of liver fibrosis or cirrhosis. In the past, a liver biopsy was required, but several non-invasive tests are now available, such as the serum FibroTest and Fibro Sure, which measure a factor in the blood indicating liver fibrosis. Also available is the FibroScan and the Shear Wave test that measure liver elasticity percutaneously.

Conventional Treatments

In the past, hepatitis C infections were treated with interferon, which had a fairly good cure rate, but also was accompanied by a number of complications, such as severe fatigue. Now most cases are treated with a group of antiviral drugs, referred to as direct-acting antiviral agents (DAAs). A combination of antiviral medications, such as elbasvir, grazoprevir, sofosbuvir, and velpatasvir are the most commonly used antiviral medications. Ribavirin is added in cases that respond poorly to conventional treatments. Side effects of the drugs, which can be troublesome, are significantly less than interferon treatments.

A cure is defined as having no detectable virus in the blood for 12 weeks and a better quality of life. Overall, for all genotypes of the virus, the cure rate is 90% and for most cases in the U.S., the cure rate is 100%.

My Recommendations

Because the damage done by these viruses is mostly caused by one's own immune reaction to the virus and not the virus itself, many innovative natural treatments are available for safe and effective treatment of both asymptomatic carriers and symptomatic individuals. In addition, several of these natural compounds also have powerful antiviral properties and can enhance the effectiveness of conventional treatments. Experimental studies indicate that several plant extracts and nutrients, described further on, can protect the liver in hepatitis B and C infections and eliminate the virus. Each works in a somewhat different way, and a combination can improve the speed and extent of recovery.

Silymarin, from milk thistle, protects the liver, but several studies found that it did not reduce the viral load (concentration of the viruses) or repair the damage to the liver by the virus. It may be that the problem in these studies was the poor absorption of raw silymarin. Nano-Silymarin, which has superior absorption and entry into cells, may have worked better. In human trials involving patients with chronic viral hepatitis, silymarin significantly reduced liver enzyme levels. And some studies have demonstrated an improvement in liver damage.

Using another type of higher absorption silymarin, researchers demonstrated a significant reduction in liver fibrosis and less progression to the cirrhosis stage. One study demonstrated that higher-absorption silymarin could prevent reinfection of transplanted livers, a major problem with liver transplants for end-stage viral hepatitis. Other studies demonstrated that silymarin could prevent transfer of infection to surrounding cells.

Vitamin E has antiviral effects and lowers liver enzymes, which is a sign of damage to the liver. An extract from green or white tea (EGCG—epigallocatechin gallate), and the teas themselves, prevent the hepatitis B virus from entering liver cells, thus preventing infection and re-infection, which can be a major problem.

Curcumin has also shown impressive results, not just in suppressing replication of the virus, but also in reducing the damage to the liver caused by the virus. Curcumin also demonstrated a reduction in infection by the hepatitis B virus by a special mechanism. Nano-Curcumin is far better absorbed and distributed to the liver.

Because of the demonstrated antiviral effects of curcumin, silymarin, quercetin, EGCG, and resveratrol, one can combine several of these natural compounds with the DAA drugs to enhance the effectiveness and safety of the conventional drugs, and in addition promote liver healing and prevent progression to liver fibrosis and cirrhosis. Curcumin has demonstrated a specific ability to suppress scarring of the liver (liver fibrosis and cirrhosis).

Studies using quercetin, a flavonoid found in higher concentrations in teas, onions, and many vegetables, has been shown to reduce the replication of hepatitis C viruses and also reduce the viral load—that is, the amount of virus in the liver and blood. Quercetin not only reduced the viral load in these studies but also reduced the ability of the virus to infect cells.

Quercetin, like curcumin, in its raw state is very poorly absorbed. Nano-Quercetin is far better absorbed from the intestines and stomach and enters the liver cells at a much higher level, where it can inhibit viral replication and survival. A combination of Nano-Curcumin and Nano-Quercetin would have an even more potent effect.

Baicalin, another plant extract, has shown very impressive results in inhibiting a number of viruses, including the hepatitis B virus. Studies demonstrate baicalin powerfully inhibits the virus from replicating, which is essential for virus infectivity. Combining baicalin with the conventional antiviral medications greatly enhances the effectiveness of these therapies and also overcomes treatment resistance. A recent study found that baicalin powerfully inhibited the growth and spread of hepatocellular carcinoma tumors as well.

Studies have shown that the hepatitis B virus can stop the immune system from defending itself, a mechanism called *immune paralysis*. Ellagic acid, extracted from plants such as pomegranates, can prevent this immune paralysis and make the virus susceptible to being killed by one's own immune system. Vitamin E also improves immunity to the hepatitis B virus.

Beta-glucan, a specific stimulant for cellular immunity, can enhance immune control of these viruses. Special immune cells (natural killer cells—NK cells and cytotoxic T cells) play a major role in viral clearance and the killing of viruses. Curcumin also stimulates these special immune cells.

Infected patients characteristically have low zinc and selenium levels, and so increasing these minerals protects the liver against damage. Vitamin C has powerful antiviral properties and reduces damage from inflammation that accompanies the disease. It should only be taken between meals to prevent iron absorption, which can enhance viral replication and liver damage. This is especially important in cases of hemochromatosis, a condition characterized by high levels of iron absorption and deposition in the liver.

Natural Supplements

Nano-Curcumin

The herb suppresses the hepatitis B and hepatitis C viruses, reduces liver inflammation and free radicals, and improves bile flow. It also inhibits liver cancer.

What to do. Take 500 to 1000 mg, three times a day with meals. This special product was designed for high absorption from the GI tract and enhanced entry into cells, especially cancer cells. Once the infection is declared cured, the Nano-Curcumin can be taken as 250 mg twice a day with a meal. Nano-Curcumin should not be taken with anticoagulant medications.

Nano-Quercetin

A nutrient found in many plants—especially teas, onions, and most vegetables—quercetin has been shown to inhibit replication of these viruses, reduce inflammation in the liver, and inhibit liver cancer development. It works best when combined with Nano-Curcumin.

What to do. Take 500 to 1000 mg three times a day with meals. This is the most absorbable form and is well tolerated. When taken on an empty stomach, it can cause hypoglycemia, which is beneficial for those with diabetes or insulin resistance, but can be a problem for those with reactive hypoglycemia. This product should be taken daily until a cure is afforded, then one can take the Nano-Quercetin, 250 mg twice a day, with a meal. It should not be combined with anticoagulant medications.

Green Tea Extract (EGCG) as Nano-EGCG

EGCG, short for epigallocatechin gallate, is the key therapeutic ingredient in green and white teas. This compound prevents hepatitis B viruses from entering liver cells and prevents the virus from replicating.

What to do. Take 100 mg, three times a day, with meals. Teavigo is a standardized, caffeine-free extract in several brands, including a product made by Pure Encapsulations. Or, drink white tea, the richest natural source of EGCG. Nano-EGCG is far better absorbed and distributed to liver cells than are plain EGCG or white tea drinks. Once the infection is cured, take the Nano-EGCG once a day with a meal. EGCG, in very rare instances, has caused liver failure itself. Stopping the compound usually returns liver functions to normal.

Ellagic Acid

Ellagic acid, a flavonoid, is a therapeutic plant compound found in higher concentrations in pomegranates, raspberries, strawberries, and walnuts. It can prevent immune paralysis, which shuts off natural defenses against the hepatitis B virus. By doing this, it makes the virus susceptible to being killed by one's immune system.

What to do. Take 300 mg, three times a day, with meals. This supplement works in conjunction with other natural compounds known to stimulate cellular immunity, such as astragalus and beta 1,3/1,6 glucan.

Nano-Silymarin

Silymarin, an extract from milk thistle, can significantly lower elevated liver enzymes, a measure of liver damage in infected people, and in studies using high-absorption forms of silymarin, can prevent viral entry into hepatocytes and lower the viral load (the number of viruses in the blood and liver). Silymarin significantly improves the histological damage to the liver by these viruses when it is adequately absorbed. It is best absorbed as the Nano-Silymarin product.

What to do. Take two 250 mg capsules of Nano-Silymarin three times a day with meals. Once a cure is determined, the Nano-Silymarin can be taken once or twice a day with a meal.

Sulforaphane

Extracted from broccoli, sulforaphane improves liver detoxification, reduces inflammation, and has been shown to inhibit cancer.

What to do. Take 400 to 800 mcg, three times a day, with meals. Swanson makes a good quality product with 400 mcg per capsule.

Pterostilbene (Resveratrol)

Found in high concentrations in grape skins and other products, resveratrol has powerful anti-inflammatory and anticancer effects and raises levels of a major internal antioxidant in our bodies: **glutathione**. Glutathione, as you have learned, plays a major role in liver protection and in detoxification. Pterostilbene is converted into resveratrol once it is absorbed and is far better absorbed than resveratrol itself.

What to do. Take 200 mg, three times daily, with a meal. Once a cure is attained, the dose can be switched to 100 mg, three times a day, with meals.

Vitamin E and Mixed Tocotrienols

In nature, vitamin E is composed of a combination of subtypes called *mixed tocopherols* and *mixed tocotrienols*. A dry form of vitamin E, which contains a major form as a succinate product, has powerful anticancer and anti-inflammatory effects. Both forms improve immunity to the virus, reduce inflammation, neutralize free radicals, and have anticancer effects. Tocotrienol has the most powerful anticancer and anti-inflammatory properties and can be taken as a separate supplement. Tocotrienol should be taken at a different time of day than the vitamin E.

What to do. Take 400 IU of mixed tocopherols or vitamin E succinate, twice a day, between meals. The dose of mixed tocotrienols is two 50 mg caplets, three times a day, with meals.

Vitamin C Buffered or Nano-Vitamin C

Vitamin C is a powerful anti-inflammatory and antioxidant, and has anticancer properties. A form called Lypo Spheric Vitamin C, made by LivOn Labs, is absorbed more effectively than regular vitamin C. It comes in packets of gel, each containing 1000 mg of vitamin C. Nano-Vitamin C is extremely well absorbed and distributed to and within cells. Vitamin C has powerful antiviral properties and prevents the cytokine storm reaction seen with overwhelming sepsis (infections).

What to do. Mix two gel packets (2000 mg) with water or juice and drink three times a day. Higher doses can be used for more serious infections. This product contains a phospholipid that in higher doses can cause muscle spasms, especially of the neck. Nano-Vitamin C comes as a 250 mg capsule. One can take three to four capsules three times a day between meals as needed. Always take vitamin C on an empty stomach, as it increases iron absorption and taking it with food can lead to excess iron levels. Iron stimulates the growth of both viral and bacterial infectious organisms.

Zinc Picolinate

Zinc levels are significantly low among people with hepatitis B and C, and with most other infections. Supplementing with zinc boosts the immune response to viral infections, and it also has antioxidant properties. Zinc picolinate is a specific high absorption form of the mineral.

What to do. Take 50 mg a day for 2 weeks, then 50 mg twice a week thereafter. For severe infections, use an initial loading dose of 300 mg.

Selenium (Selenomethionine)

This mineral plays a major role in immune function and is essential for important internal detoxification processes in our bodies. In addition, it has significant anticancer properties. Selenomethionine, available in several brands of supplements, is a form that is especially well absorbed.

What to do. Take 200 mcg a day for 3 days and then reduce the dose to 100 mcg a day. It can be taken long-term for general health in a dose of 100 mcg a day with food.

Branched Chain Amino Acids

Called BCAAs for short, these are three specific building blocks of protein: leucine, isoleucine, and valine. A number of studies have shown that they protect the liver and promote its healing. This amino acid combination can trigger hypoglycemia, especially in individuals having reactive hypoglycemia, so it should always be taken with meals.

What to do. Take approximately 3 grams of a powder (between a half and one scoop, depending on the product), mixed with water or juice, with a meal. Only the micronized form is water soluble, and it is far better absorbed.

Fish Oil

In all cases of hepatitis, levels of omega-3 fatty acid are very low, which makes the liver highly susceptible to inflammation and viral damage. Several studies have shown that the omega-3 fats in fish oil reduce liver inflammation and help protect liver cells from viral damage. The best form to take is DHA, not the high EPA form. High EPA can thin the blood, resulting in hemorrhages in some people. DHA is the major form used in the body to reduce inflammation and heal the liver. DHA levels are extremely low in cases of hepatitis. Supplementation with omega-3 fatty acids has been shown to reduce the level of inflammatory cytokines in the liver, thus improving liver function. In addition, DHA has been shown to increase the killing of liver cancer cells.

What to do. Take pure DHA or at least a form that is mostly DHA, and no more than 170 mg of EPA per caplet or capsule. The dose to take is between 1000 and 2000 mg of DHA a day, taken with food. DHA should be kept in the refrigerator.

CHAPTER 13

Fatty Liver Disease

The Silent Killer

O ften called the "silent" liver disease, this condition is on the rise, and has replaced excessive alcohol consumption as the most common cause of liver disease.

In the U.S., it has become a leading cause for liver transplants.

The main danger of fatty liver disease is that, in its earlier stages, it rarely causes any symptoms until it damages the liver, and by then significant damage may have occurred.

Fatty Liver Disease

Fatty liver disease falls into two categories; nonalcoholic fatty liver disease, or NAFLD, and nonalcoholic steatohepatitis, or NASH.

Nonalcoholic fatty liver disease, or NAFLD, is a buildup of extra fat cells in the liver. In this condition, fat accumulates in the liver but alcohol is not a contributing factor.

The liver is considered fatty if more than 5 to 10% of its weight is comprised of fat. Between 10 and 20% of Americans have nonalcoholic liver disease.

With nonalcoholic steatohepatitis, or NASH, fat in the liver is accompanied by inflammation, which damages the liver. As liver cells die, they are replaced by scar tissue (liver fibrosis), and, if the scarring progresses far enough, it reaches the stage of cirrhosis. At this point, we can see liver failure. It's estimated that 5 to 10% of people with fatty liver disease go on to develop NASH.

People with NASH can remain stable for years, experiencing no or few symptoms, but in an estimated 3 to 26% of people, the disease can cause serious liver damage. The presence of inflammation and scarring can result in the need for a liver transplant. NASH is also linked to liver cancer. Liver cancer with NAFLD, however, is rare.

Up until a few years ago, most people who needed new livers were those with hepatitis C. But with today's progress in treatments, the cure rate for hepatitis C has risen to 95%, so the focus is on NASH and other causes for liver inflammation.

NASH, as stated, ultimately causes cirrhosis, an ailment traditionally associated with alcoholics. Although NASH occurs in nondrinkers, the disease process is basically the same.

However, even if the condition is only NAFLD, this is a serious sign of increased risk of heart disease, diabetes, and other metabolic disorders, and needs to be addressed.

There are no pharmaceutical medications that correct or reverse any type of fatty liver disease. Diet, exercise, weight loss, and avoidance of any unnecessary medications are today's current treatment. A number of natural products can also reduce fatty liver pathology and prevent progression to NASH, liver fibrosis, and cirrhosis. If the condition progresses to a point of liver failure, a liver transplant is the only option. The best option is to not let things reach that point.

There is a move to replace the term "nonalcoholic fatty liver disease" with "metabolic fatty liver disease," because this term more accurately describes the cause of the condition.

Fatty Liver Disease Symptoms

Fatty liver disease is known as a "silent killer" because it does not generally cause symptoms. When it does, the symptoms, such as abdominal discomfort, weakness, or fatigue, are usually brushed aside or ascribed to other conditions. Even if the disease progresses to NASH, no symptoms may occur until the liver damage becomes serious.

Symptoms of Fatty Liver Disease

In most cases, there are few if any symptoms of abnormal fat in the liver, but when it's accompanied by inflammation and liver damage, initial damage can include fatigue, weakness, right upper quadrant abdominal pain, and weight loss. As with cirrhosis, severe scarring and hardening of the liver interferes with normal liver function, causing the following:

- Swollen belly (fluid retention)
- Yellowish skin and eyes (jaundice)
- Intestinal bleeding
- Muscle wasting
- Liver cancer
- Liver failure

Risk Factors for NAFLD and NASH

Obesity

Obesity and being overweight is the major cause of NAFLD, and it is the obesity crisis that is fueling the rise of this condition, including in young people. Fatty liver disease is 7 to 10 times more common in the obese. Of importance is the fact that the most common causes for the obesity epidemic is a dramatic increase in consuming excitotoxin-containing foods (MSG, hydrolyzed proteins, soy protein isolates, etc.) and an equally dramatic increase in the consumption of high-fructose corn syrup.

Obesity causes chronic bodily inflammation, which is a form of smoldering inflammation you cannot feel, but is a major cause of chronic disease, including NAFLD.

There is no test that can accurately predict which people with NAFLD will develop NASH, but it is known that the following risk factors ratchet up the risk.

Gender

Traditionally, men have been at higher risk for NAFLD and NASH. However, some research is finding that when women do develop NAFLD, they are at higher risk of it progressing, and some studies indicate that women may also be at a higher risk after menopause. A review of 60 studies, published in 2020 in the journal *Endocrinology*, found this to be true for both NAFLD and NASH, but the risk was low for women of normal weight, glucose, and insulin levels.

Heredity

Fatty liver disease is not strictly inherited, but there is a form of NASH that can occur more often in families. Talk to your doctor if NASH has occurred either on your mother's or father's side of the family. If you have a genetic predisposition to NASH, it may not matter whether or not you are overweight. Also, it is important to keep in mind that the strongest link to NASH is abdominal obesity, which can, in some instances, occur in thin people.

Diabetes

Type 2 diabetes (the most common form of diabetes) or insulin resistance, which can occur prior to this condition, is a risk factor for NAFLD. This is because, when muscle, liver, and fat cells don't respond properly to insulin, this results in an increase of the amount of free fatty acids in the blood. Some of these fat molecules may accumulate in the liver, resulting in inflammation induced liver damage. Inflammation increases fatty acid accumulation by fat cells.

Metabolic Syndrome

This term refers to a cluster of conditions that significantly increases the risk for fatty liver disease, including the propensity of developing NASH. People are said to have metabolic syndrome if they have three or more of these conditions: abdominal obesity, high triglycerides, insulin resistance, glucose intolerance, and high blood pressure. Metabolic syndrome also leads to inflammation, which is believed a key contributor to fatty liver disease and NASH. Metabolic syndrome is strongly linked to type 2 diabetes.

There are also less common risk factors for NAFLD and NASH. These include:

- **Obstructive sleep apnea.** A common sleep disorder. Its connection with NAFLD is explored later in this chapter.
- **Polycystic ovary syndrome.** A condition in women that is characterized by irregular or no menstrual periods, acne, obesity, and excessive hair growth. It affects 5 to 10% of

women of reproductive age. This syndrome is linked to insulin resistance.

- **Underactive thyroid (hypothyroidism).** The thyroid gland controls metabolism. An underactive thyroid causes your metabolism to slow down, leading to an accumulation of fat in your body, which increases the risk of developing NAFLD.
- **Lipid storage diseases.** This is a group of hereditary metabolic disorders that cause harmful fatty materials to accumulate in various cells and tissues of several organs, including the liver.
- **Rapid weight loss.** Weight loss can help reverse fatty liver disease, but research finds that if this is done too rapidly, it can actually worsen the condition. Weight loss of no more than a few pounds a week is best.
- **Hepatitis C.**
- **Exposure to some toxic substances.**

Certain drugs also raise the risk, such as the following:

- Amiodarone
- Diltiazem
- Glucocorticoids
- Highly active antiretroviral therapy
- Methotrexate
- Synthetic estrogens
- Tamoxifen
- Valproic acid

SIBO

The condition known as small intestinal bacterial overgrowth (SIBO) is linked to the development of fatty liver disease.

Fatty Liver Disease—The High-Fructose Corn Syrup Connection

There is a strong connection between the increasing consumption of high-fructose corn syrup and these liver disorders.

Back in the early 1900s, refined sugar played a minor role in our diet. Americans consumed a very modest amount of sugar, only a fraction of the amount we consume today.

But, in addition to the higher amount of sugar we consume today, another major change took place in 1970, when high-fructose corn syrup (HFCS) was introduced into our food supply due to rising cane and beet sugar costs. HFCS was quickly adopted by the food industry.

Our body handles fructose and glucose in different ways. Virtually any cell in our body can utilize glucose, but only liver cells metabolize fructose.

Refined sugar (sucrose) is comprised of two sugar molecules: one of fructose and one of glucose. But HFCS contains more fructose: 55% compared to 45% glucose.

This means that the liver must handle a higher amount of fructose, which is metabolized into fat. If there is too much fructose, tiny droplets of fat form in the liver.

Fatty liver disease was unknown until about 1980 and many experts—myself included—believe that its occurrence, at around the time manufacturers were shifting to the use of HFCS, is no coincidence.

Unfortunately, HFCS has crept into almost all manufactured and processed foods—even those that don't taste sweet, such as frozen vegetables or salad dressings—so the easiest way to avoid it is to limit your intake of these items and stick to whole foods most of the time. Here are some guidelines:

- Choose fresh organic whole produce, such as fresh fruits and vegetables.
- Eliminate processed foods and foods containing added sugar.
- Avoid sodas (both sweetened and artificially sweetened, as well as processed fruit); choose purified water or tea instead.
- Snack on foods such as nuts. Use only limited amounts in snacking.

What's Your Gut Bacteria Got to Do with Fatty Liver Disease?

The study of gut bacteria is a relatively new field of science that is producing many answers to long-standing questions about chronic diseases, including those that affect the liver.

You know that bacteria can cause illness, but research now shows that our gut contains trillions of microorganisms, including at least 1000 known species of bacteria. These include so-called good bacteria that are responsible for many of our body's necessary functions, including digestion, and that the composition of these bacteria, known as our "gut microbiota," differs from individual to individual, yet is stable in most individuals for a lifetime. However, use of antibiotics and other medications harmful to gut bacteria can cause their balance to change over time.

Science is discovering many fascinating things about our microbiota. For instance, one study showed that a certain type of gut bacteria, known as *K. pneumonia*, produces a large amount of alcohol, even in nondrinkers. The study found that this common form of bacteria, which is not considered harmful, was found in over 60% of NAFLD patients and only 6% of the healthy control subjects.

"These bacteria damage your liver just like alcohol, except you don't have a choice," said Jing Yuan, lead author of the study, which was published in the journal *Cell Metabolism*.

It is unknown why some people have a high-alcohol-producing *K. pneumonia* strain in their gut, while others don't, but the researchers don't believe this type of bacteria is extremely common, otherwise the rates of NAFLD would be even higher. They also surmised that the reason might be that some people have a gut microbiome that is more favorable to this type of bacteria, which allows it to flourish.

Gut bacteria also play a major role in controlling inflammation, anywhere in the body—even in the liver and brain. Several probiotics of the lactobacillus and bifidobacteria reduce inflammation.

SIBO and NAFLD

Small intestinal bacterial overgrowth (SIBO) is defined as the presence of an abnormally high number of coliform bacteria in the small bowel, which can cause symptoms such as bloating. Research finds that people with NAFLD are also more likely to have SIBO as well.

Sleep Apnea and Fatty Liver Disease

Obstructive sleep apnea is a common sleep disorder that occurs when your throat muscles intermittently relax and block your airway, in some people hundreds of times a night.

Sleep apnea is a contributor to many chronic diseases, including heart disease, high blood pressure, stroke, diabetes, sudden cardiac death, and others, as well as fatty liver disease.

Studies have found that this type of sleep apnea, which results in oxidative stress, as well as periodic low oxygen levels, can worsen nonalcoholic fatty liver disease and may even tip its progression into NASH. There is a very strong link between sleep apnea and inflammation, which explains its link to obesity. Some studies have shown that surgical removal of abdominal fat can cure a high percentage of cases of sleep apnea. Dietary control is a better option, however.

There are treatment options available for sleep apnea, which include the CPAP (Continuous Positive Airway Pressure Device), as well as others, which are surgically implanted.

The primary symptom of sleep apnea is loud snoring. Other symptoms include:

- Excessive daytime sleepiness, which can lead to accidents during the day
- Abrupt awakening accompanied by shortness of breath
- Awakening with a dry mouth or sore throat
- Awakening coughing or gagging
- Morning headache
- Difficulty staying asleep
- Problems paying attention or focusing

Although sleep apnea is often considered a problem in men, women can develop it as well. Sometimes women snore loudly, but their other symptoms may be subtler and include:

- Light snoring
- Subtle breathing difficulties
- Awakening with a dry mouth
- Falling asleep only to wake up almost immediately.

If you think you may have sleep apnea, ask your doctor for a referral to a reputable sleep clinic.

The NAFLD–MSG Connection

Current research also suggests that modern diets are the main culprit in NAFLD. In most cases, if the diet is changed, the condition can improve and even be eliminated.

Dr. Kate Collison, a researcher at the Cell Biology & Diabetes Research Unit, Department of Biological Sciences, in Saudi Arabia, shared with me some of her groundbreaking research on this subject.

Dr. Collison's research clearly shows that a combination of a high intake of trans fats (partially hydrogenated oils such as corn, safflower, sunflower, peanut, and soybean oils), along with monosodium glutamate (MSG), leads to liver damage as well as metabolic syndrome, obesity, type 2 diabetes, and insulin resistance.

MSG alone has been shown to produce intense storms of free radicals and lipid peroxidation products in the liver, an organ that is especially at risk because the blood from the intestines and colon drains directly into the liver, creating high concentrations of toxic substances.

Interestingly, trans fatty acids, high-fructose corn syrup, and MSG all raised cholesterol levels, produced insulin resistance, and caused fat to accumulate in the abdomen (called *visceral fat*).

How Fatty Liver Disease Damages Your Heart

Cardiovascular disease (heart attack and stroke) is the most common cause of death in people with fatty liver disease, so no matter what form of this disease you have, you need to be concerned about its impact on your heart.

Although NASH can be fatal, this serious disease affects a minority of people with fatty liver disease. The most common causes of death for people with fatty liver disease are cardiovascular and cerebrovascular disease, which encompasses both heart attacks and strokes (cerebrovascular disease).

Although the exact mechanism of this connection between heart health and fatty liver disease isn't known for certain, there is compelling evidence that the link is inflammation, which has been shown to be the primary mechanism for atherosclerosis and heart disease. Because people developing fatty liver disease are more prone to develop the following heart problems, they should be monitored by their health care professionals. These conditions include:

- **Coronary heart disease.** The narrowing of the heart's coronary arteries, which sets the stage for heart attack. When this occurs in the blood vessels supplying the brain, it can cause a stroke.
- **Left ventricular hypertrophy.** An enlargement and weakening of the heart's main pumping chamber, which is an independent predictor for coronary heart disease, sudden death, heart failure, and stroke.
- **Increased fat within the heart.** This condition occurs with aging and is an indicator of serious coronary heart disease. This is a commonly ignored disorder.
- **Damage to the heart valves**, including aortic stenosis and mitral valve calcification, both of which prevent the heart from functioning properly.
- **Cardiac arrhythmias** (such as atrial fibrillation and ventricular fibrillation), as well as electrical conduction defects, such as heart blockages of varying degrees, which can lead to heart attacks.

How to Heal Fatty Liver Disease

Currently, there is no medical treatments for nonalcoholic fatty liver disease, but it can be prevented, or, if caught at an early stage, possibly reversed. Here's how to do that:

- **Lose weight.** Losing even 10% of your weight can reduce your risk.
- **Exercise daily.** For instance, a study in 2020 demonstrated the benefits of aerobic exercise on people with NAFLD. All exercise is helpful.
- **Eliminate all foods containing sugar,** which includes candy, pies, and cake, but also other "hidden" sugar as well, which can be found in processed and packaged foods. Choose organic whole foods instead.
- **Avoid artificial sweeteners,** especially aspartame, saccharin, and Splenda.
- **Eliminate fried foods** and any food cooked with or using omega-6 oils.
- **Eliminate MSG** and all excitotoxin food additives (natural flavoring, hydrolyzed proteins, soy protein extracts or isolates, autolyzed yeast, carrageenan, broth, etc.).
- **Cut out foods containing high-fructose corn syrup,** which may be fueling the fatty liver disease epidemic because it converts more quickly to fat and promotes inflammation. (See the recommendations earlier.)
- **Eat lots of steamed cruciferous veggies.** Recent research finds that indole-3 carbinol, a natural compound found in many vegetables, may help decrease fat and inflammation in the liver. Cruciferous vegetables include cabbage, kale, cauliflower, and Brussels sprouts.
- **Avoid all unnecessary medications** that stress the liver when possible (warnings on labels should indicate this).

- **Avoid all sources of fluoride.** Found in dried fruits (especially raisins), public drinking water, black tea, etc. Use a filter to remove fluoride from your drinking water or drink distilled water.
- **Dietary fats do not directly cause liver disease.** However, omega-6 oils, such as corn, safflower, sunflower, peanut, and soybean oils, should be avoided, because these increase inflammation in the liver and all tissues and organs.
- **Drink white or green teas.** Several studies find that catechin in these not only aids in weight loss, but also reduces inflammation and other factors that may help reduce fat in the liver.

Some research shows that people with fatty liver disease may not be able to metabolize iron sufficiently, leading to a lesser ability to exercise, so in this case diet becomes more important.

Supplements

The following supplements protect your liver and heal the damage of NAFLD:

Silymarin (as Nano-Silymarin)

An extract made from milk thistle, silymarin has been shown to protect liver cells, reduce inflammation, prevent liver scarring, and inhibit liver cancer. Silymarin is normally poorly absorbed. The Nano-Silymarin form, made by One Planet Nutrition Company, is very well absorbed and distributed in the liver.

What to do. Take one or two 250 mg capsules of the Nano-Silymarin three times a day with meals.

Curcumin (as Nano-Curcumin)

This herbal extract reduces liver inflammation, is an antioxidant, promotes bile flow, inhibits liver cancer growth and invasion, and inhibits fat accumulation in fat cells (thus reducing fatty liver disease). Curcumin is very poorly absorbed in its natural form. The Nano-Curcumin product, made by One Planet Nutrition Company, is very well absorbed and distributed in the liver.

What to do. Take one 250 mg capsule, three times a day, with meals.

Quercetin (as Nano-Quercetin)

Has been shown to be particularly protective of the liver, especially when used in conjunction with curcumin. The dose is one 250 mg capsule twice to three times a day with meals. It is also a significant inhibitor of liver cancer.

N-acetyl-L-cysteine

Plays an important role in increasing cellular levels of the powerful antioxidant glutathione. It is also an important chelator (binder) of toxic metals. It is best taken with a meal.

What to do. The usual dose is 500 to 900 mg taken once or twice a day with food.

Baicalin

This natural compound has been shown to reduce fat accumulation by the liver, reduce free radical damage, potently reduce inflammation, inhibit liver cancer, and remove toxic levels of iron from the liver.

What to do. The usual dose of baicalin is 250 mg taken twice a day. If you want to remove excess iron, it should be taken with meals. If you have no iron problems, it should be taken at least 45 minutes before a meal and with buffered vitamin C in a dose of 500 mg.

Hesperidin

This natural flavonoid has been shown to significantly protect the liver from fat infiltration and prevent liver fibrosis. It also reduces obesity, reduces inflammation, reduces liver fibrosis, is a powerful antioxidant, prevents liver cancer, and inhibits atherosclerosis.

What to do. The dose is 500 mg taken three times a day with meals.

DHA (from Omega-3 Oils)

DHA is a component extracted from omega-3 oils. Studies have shown that omega-3 oils, especially DHA, are depleted from cirrhotic livers. DHA has powerful anti-inflammatory effects, reduces the risk of cancer, and is vital for the functioning of all cells.

What to do. The best effects are seen with products having at least 70% DHA or even pure DHA of the triglyceride form. The dose is 1000 mg taken twice to three times a day with meals.

Magnesium citrate/malate

Increases liver cell glutathione, reduces inflammation, improves blood flow, and prevents gallstones. The slow-release form of magnesium citrate/malate is best in terms of the absorption and prevention of diarrhea. The Jigsaw Health company makes a slow release form.

What to do. Take two tablets twice a day with a meal.

Vitamin D$_3$

This is an immune modulator, which means it reduces inflammation. It also boosts resistance to infections and has many other protective functions. Most people have moderate to severe deficiencies of this critical vitamin. A vitamin D$_3$ level test should be done before supplementing. The optimal levels of vitamin D$_3$ ranges from 65 ng/ml to 100 ng/ml. Those with high calcium levels should take this vitamin under the direction of a physician trained in this area. Severe vitamin D$_3$ deficiency is very common in the elderly, especially institutionalized elderly.

What to do. Studies have shown that blood levels are not increased until one takes at least 2000 IU a day. Most authorities suggest 5000 IU a day with food. Studies have shown that taking vitamin D$_3$ daily is superior to taking a larger dose once a week.

Taurine

A sulfur-containing amino acid that is essential for liver detoxification. Taurine is also a neuromodulator and neurotransmitter for the brain. Several studies have shown it can correct several types of arrhythmias and improve heart function.

What to do. The dose is 500 to 1000 mg, twice to three times a day, taken 30 minutes before meals.

Berberine

Berberine is a natural plant extract that has shown a great number of beneficial effects, including being an anti-inflammatory, an antioxidant, and reducing fat accumulation in the liver. One study involving 184 patients with NAFLD demonstrated a highly significant effect of berberine in removing fat from the liver and preventing progression to worse liver diseases in those taking berberine. Berberine also significantly lowered elevated blood sugar and corrected abnormal lipid profiles.

What to do. The dose of berberine used in this study was 500 mg taken three times a day with meals.

Important Note: I'm often asked if it is necessary to take all these supplements. The answer is no. One should take basic vitamins and minerals and then use the more powerful compounds for more serious cases. For example, one can start with the basics: DHA, vitamin D$_3$, vitamin E (mixed tocopherols), B-complex vitamins, vitamin C buffered, and magnesium. Use one of the other compounds as needed. For instance, one can start with Nano-Curcumin for 3 weeks. If more is needed, add taurine. The third compound to try might be the berberine. Products are added as needed, giving at least 3 weeks for each to see if more is required.

Future Research

At present, there is no traditional medical cure or pharmaceutical treatment for NAFLD, but research is ongoing. Even though the best results presently are with natural treatments. Every year we learn a great deal more about how the liver functions and a great deal more about these diseases themselves. Parallel with this growth of knowledge, we are learning a great deal concerning each of these natural compounds and how they can interact with what we are discovering about the pathophysiology of these diseases. The study of nutrition and the use of natural compounds is far outdistancing pharmaceutical drugs in terms of safety and effectiveness.

CHAPTER 14

Cirrhosis of the Liver

Cirrhosis is a pathological process that generally follows a specific set of steps. While cirrhosis is by far the most dangerous nonmalignant process affecting the liver, it does not always occur in liver damaging disorders. For example, cirrhosis is very rare in cases of nonalcoholic fatty liver diseases (NAFLD), but more common with nonalcoholic steatohepatitis (NASH) and viral hepatitis caused by type C and B hepatitis viruses, especially type C viral hepatitis. Approximately 20% of hepatitis C cases and 10% of NASH cases will progress to cirrhosis.

In the cases where the damage becomes progressive, the first stage is liver fibrosis, in which scar tissue (collagen) begins to build up in the lobules of the liver. At this stage, the liver's function is somewhat impaired but, overall, still functioning well enough for general health. As the scar tissue continues to build, other changes occur that further impair liver function, such as dense fibrous bands and regenerative nodules that begin to appear, and processes that not only result in the death of the liver's main cells, the hepatocytes, but also interfere with the blood drainage system of the liver, called the *hepatic portal system*. This system of veins travels from the intestines to the liver and is also linked to the kidneys, esophagus, and stomach.

When this venous system is blocked, we begin to see massive amounts of fluid accumulate in the abdomen (called *ascites*), which can take on the appearance of a hugely swollen belly. The obstruction of the veins around the lower esophagus take on the appearance of hemorrhoids (called *variceal veins*). These thin-walled veins are subject to sudden rupturing, leading to massive bleeding into the esophagus and stomach. Obstruction of this venous system also impairs kidney function and can result in rapid death.

Cirrhosis is the most common form of advanced chronic liver disease. In many cases, the advanced stage of liver scarring can take decades to fully develop, all depending on the causative agent. Chronic viral liver damage can take much longer to develop into cirrhosis than many types of chemical damage, such as we see with exposure to carbon tetrachloride, which can destroy the liver in a matter of hours.

It has been estimated that approximately 1% of the U.S. population has cirrhosis, but many cases are never suspected during the life of the individual and are only discovered during autopsies. Many unsuspected cases are also discovered during routine laboratory screenings.

In many cases, we see preexisting liver damage of some degree before cirrhosis develops. For example, a person who drinks alcohol moderately will be more susceptible to severe liver damage by viral hepatitis than would a healthy abstainer. The same would be true for those who use aspartame regularly or acetaminophen. Both of these compounds cause variable degrees of damage to the liver and deplete the liver's glutathione content, one of its most important antioxidant protectants.

Being male and being older in age also increase one's risk of developing cirrhosis following infections with the hepatitis C virus.

Heredity can also play a role, because some people are born with deficient levels of liver protectants or detoxification enzymes.

In the Western world, alcoholic liver disease and hepatitis C virus are the most common cause of cirrhosis. Hepatitis B is the most common cause in Asia and sub-Saharan areas. In 1998, in the U.S., there were 25,000 deaths attributed to cirrhosis and 373,000 hospitalizations.

Complications associated with cirrhosis include variceal hemorrhage, ascites, spontaneous bacterial peritonitis, and hepatic encephalopathy. These complications signal impending death unless a liver transplant is done quickly.

Major Causes of Cirrhosis

Hepatitis C

Hepatitis C is the most common cause of cirrhosis, slightly edging out chronic alcohol abuse. Hepatitis B and D can cause cirrhosis as well, but hepatitis C is the far more common cause.

Chronic Alcohol Abuse

About 10 to 20% of heavy drinkers develop cirrhosis. According to the National Institute on Drug Abuse and Alcoholism, heavy drinking is defined as drinking five or more drinks in one day on at least five of the previous 30 days. But alcoholic cirrhosis is not confined to heavy drinkers. A study in 2008 demonstrated that even moderate levels of alcohol consumption increase the risk of cirrhosis. The study also found that the risk for cirrhosis was higher in people who drank alcohol during times other than meals, or who drank daily.

Regular use of other liver toxic substances, such as aspartame, acetaminophen, exposure to industrial chemicals, pesticides, and herbicides, and some prescription drugs also greatly increases the risk of alcohol-induced cirrhosis.

Nonalcoholic Fatty Liver Disease (NAFLD)

This is a very rare cause of cirrhosis, because most cases are not associated with significant liver damage. When such cases *are* connected, with progression to NASH and liver fibrosis, other factors are usually involved, such as alcohol abuse, obesity, undiagnosed viral hepatitis, exposure to liver toxic chemicals, and older age, especially among frail elderly individuals. The risk in healthy elderly, even at the extremes of age, is negligible.

Lesser Causes of Cirrhosis

- Iron buildup in the body (hemochromatosis)
- Cystic fibrosis
- Copper accumulated in the liver (Wilson's disease)
- Poorly formed bile ducts (biliary atresia)
- Alpha-1 antitrypsin deficiency
- Inherited disorders of sugar metabolism (galactosemia or glycogen storage disease)
- Genetic digestive disorder (Alagille syndrome)
- Liver disease caused by your body's immune system (autoimmune hepatitis)
- Destruction of the bile ducts (primary biliary cirrhosis)
- Hardening and scarring of the bile ducts (primary sclerosing cholangitis)
- Infection, such as syphilis or brucellosis
- Medications, including methotrexate or isoniazid

Risk Factors for Different Types of Cirrhosis

Excessive Alcohol Consumption

There is a myth that all cirrhosis is the result of heavy drinking. While alcohol abuse is a major cause of cirrhosis, it is not the only condition that can cause this form of liver damage. Another myth about alcohol and cirrhosis is that only heavy drinkers develop it, but some people's livers are more sensitive to the effect of alcohol. In most such cases, a poor diet or abuse of drugs is involved.

Once liver damage is detected, continued use of alcohol will result in even more rapid decompensation of the liver, leading to advanced cirrhosis. Once liver decompensation occurs, mortality rises to 85% over 5 years.

In many cases, liver function will worsen after the alcohol is stopped because alcohol is immunosuppressive and stopping it will result in an overreaction of the immune system within the liver, causing additional damage. This is controlled with steroids.

Several natural products can reduce the liver damage and prevent the hyperimmune reaction. This includes vitamin D_3, vitamin K, Nano-Curcumin, Nano-Quercetin, and Nano-Silymarin.

Obesity

Being obese or overweight increases your risk of developing conditions that lead to cirrhosis, including nonalcoholic fatty liver disease (NAFLD) and nonalcoholic steatohepatitis (NASH). Obesity is strongly associated with the metabolic syndrome, type 2 diabetes, and insulin resistance, all on the basis of stimulating chronic inflammation.

Obesity, based on its link to chronic inflammation, is strongly linked to hepatocellular carcinoma of the liver and to pancreatic cancer, both very deadly cancers with a five-year survival of only 4 to 8%. In fact, obesity makes a stronger contribution to the risk of developing hepatocellular cancer than does having hepatitis B or hepatitis C infections. Another link to obesity is the high incidence of type 2 diabetes, which is also strongly linked to the risk of hepatocellular cancer.

When you combine obesity with alcohol use, smoking, and the use of oral contraceptives, the risk for developing these cancers rises much higher.

Viral Hepatitis

Not everyone with chronic hepatitis develops cirrhosis, but having this disease does raise your risk. As discussed earlier, any condition that damages the liver, such as NAFLD, NASH, use of alcohol, use of artificial sweeteners (aspartame), regular acetaminophen use, obesity, diabetes, exposure to pesticides, herbicides, or industrial chemicals, and a poor diet, can greatly worsen the damaging effects of viral hepatitis or any other cause of liver damage.

Cirrhosis and Gender

Generally, men are twice as likely as women to die of cirrhosis. However, women are also at risk because they don't have as many enzymes in their stomach to break down alcohol. Because of this, more alcohol will reach the liver and induce scar tissue.

Cirrhosis and Age

Older people are generally thought of as the ones most likely to develop cirrhosis. Nevertheless, symptoms of alcoholic cirrhosis can develop between the ages of 30 and 40, and not become noticeable until the disease progresses.

People are also developing alcoholic cirrhosis at younger ages. A study that tracked deaths from cirrhosis over a 10-year period showed that deaths jumped by 65% in the 25- to 34-year age group, with the increase being fueled mostly by deaths due to alcohol.

With advances in age, we see a decline in the efficiency of the detoxification enzymes and protective antioxidant enzymes and glutathione, all of which puts these individuals at a higher risk of liver damage from any cause. A proper diet and the use of selected nutritional supplements and flavonoids can significantly restore liver function in the aged.

Symptoms of Cirrhosis

In some people, there are no early symptoms, so their illness only becomes apparent after the liver is badly damaged. Here are some signs that may occur earlier:

- Feeling tired or weak
- Easily bleeding or bruising
- Losing weight without trying
- Loss of appetite
- Nausea and vomiting
- Mild pain or discomfort
- Swelling in the legs, feet, or ankles (edema)
- Itchy skin
- Yellow discoloration in the skin and eyes (jaundice)
- Fluid accumulation in the abdomen (ascites)
- Spider-like blood vessels on the skin
- Redness in the palms of the hands

- For women, absent periods or a complete loss of them, unrelated to menopause
- For men, loss of sex drive, breast enlargement (gynecomastia), or testicular atrophy
- Confusion, drowsiness, and slurred speech (early hepatic encephalopathy)

In more advanced cases of cirrhosis of the liver, there can occur bleeding from the esophagus and stomach (vomiting black or dark red blood), tight swollen abdomen (ascites), sudden inflammation in the abdomen (bacterial peritonitis), an increased incidence of bacterial infections, widespread inflammation affecting many body parts, and as liver function further declines, hepatic encephalopathy.

Hepatic encephalopathy is one of the more dangerous signs of liver decompensation and can progress to stupor and coma very quickly. Death soon follows a coma.

In about 10 to 20% of cases, we see what is called the *hepatopulmonary syndrome*, a condition in which there is an overproduction of nitric oxide in the pulmonary arteries, which can lead to severe depressed oxygen levels (hypoxemia). And in 16 to 20% of patients with ascites, we see a dangerous elevation in pulmonary blood pressure (portopulmonary hypertension). These are all signs of rapid decompensation of liver function, requiring emergency treatments.

In the past, it was assumed that cirrhosis was a progressive disorder and always terminated with a need for a liver transplant. Newer studies now indicate that several treatments can reverse this process, returning the liver to more normal functions. In one such study of 153 biopsy proven cases of cirrhosis, researchers found that in 75 cases a reversal of the damage occurred after treatment of the causes. This shows the liver has a greater ability to regenerate itself than any other organ in the body.

Many natural compounds have been found to dramatically protect the liver from damage and either stop the progression of liver disease or even reverse it.

Diagnosis

The diagnosis of cirrhosis generally includes the following tests:

Laboratory Tests

Liver enzymes (transaminases), when elevated, are some of the earliest indicators of liver malfunction, but even in cases of cirrhosis, liver enzymes can be normal or only slightly elevated for long periods. Because the liver plays a major role in blood clotting, a test called the *international normalized ratio* (INR) will be checked to see if your blood is clotting properly. Serum albumin is also done to evaluate the ability of the liver to produce this important blood protein.

Imaging Tests

Ultrasounds, MRI scans, and CT scans may not be sensitive enough to fully diagnose cirrhosis, but they *can* lead to further suspicions of its existence. The ultrasound may show the typical shrinkage (atrophy) of the right lobe of the liver and enlargement (hypertrophy) of the left lobe. The MRI and CT scans cannot define the severity of the cirrhosis, but a helical MRI with contrast can detect liver cancer or vascular conditions of the liver.

The MRI scan can detect excess iron in the liver, as we see with hemochromatosis, and an excess of fat in the liver associated with fatty liver disorders (NAFLD and NASH).

Magnetic resonance elastography (MRE) may be recommended. The **FibroScan** determines the elasticity of the liver, which is lost with advanced cirrhosis. The **Shear Wave** test uses pulse ultrasound to determine liver fibrosis. The advantage is that these are non-invasive tests not requiring surgery or needle biopsy.

Biopsy

A liver biopsy is considered the gold standard for diagnosis, as it allows direct determination of the degree of fibrosis and the grade of histologic damage. Cirrhosis is divided into four grades of damage. A tissue sample (biopsy) is not necessarily needed for diagnosis and can be dangerous. Advanced cirrhosis is associated with coagulation problems and severe bleeding during a biopsy occurs in 2 to 3% of cases. Most bleeding complications occur within 24 hours of the biopsy. Your doctor may choose a biopsy to identify the severity, extent, and cause of liver damage.

Prognosis Determination

Experts in liver disorders use two main systems to determine prognosis of cirrhosis, the Child-Pugh-Turotte (CPT) classification and the MELD (Model for End Stage Liver Disease) system. The CPT system predicts development of complications and is divided into A, B, and C classes, based on a one-year survival prediction. Class A has a 100% one-year survival, class B an 80% one-year survival, and class C a 45% one-year survival.

The MELD system is more precise and predicts the best 3-month survival no matter the etiology. The score is based on the creatinine and bilirubin, plus INR. This test also detects which patients are more likely to die without a liver transplant.

Hepatic Encephalopathy

One of the most devastating late-stage effects of liver destruction is damage to the brain, which occurs in stages, from mild to severe (coma). Brain effects of liver disease do not necessarily mean that the liver destruction is advanced, because mild hepatic encephalopathy can occur rather subtly. More severe cases can severely impair brain function and lead to coma, which occurs just before death.

Hepatic encephalopathy can occur as a result of cirrhosis or can follow porto-systemic shunting operations. Other associated factors can also cause mental problems, such as associated infections, kidney failure, use of drugs, and preexisting neuro-psychiatric problems. Of these, the most strongly linked to brain impairment are infections. Cognitive impairment is seen in 42% of patients with no infections, 79% of patients with an infection, and 90% of patients with severe infections (sepsis).

Impairment of mental function is classified according to the severity of the mental problem by the West Haven Criteria.

Grade 1
- Minor lack of awareness
- Euphoria or anxiety
- Short attention span
- Impaired ability to do addition or subtraction

Grade 2
- Lethargy or apathy
- Personality change
- Disoriented in time
- Inappropriate behavior

Grade 3

- Somnolence or semi-stupor
- Confusion
- Gross disorientation

Grade 4

- Coma

Unfortunately, most doctors treating these patients have ignored minimal hepatic encephalopathy problems. While most of the symptoms are considered minor, they can interfere with one's quality of life. One can experience the following:

- Sleep disturbances
- Falls
- Poor driving ability (frequent car accidents)
- Problems with employment
- Adverse effects on survival

A number of special tests are used to detect mental impairment, such as an EEG, scan test, Clicker-Flicker frequency test (CFF), and a psychometric hepatic encephalopathy test.

How liver cirrhosis actually causes brain function to falter is debated, but there is strong evidence that inflammation in the liver activates inflammation-producing immune cells in the brain called **microglia**, and these cells, when activated, release both inflammatory compounds and excitotoxins, which together damage brain cells—especially in the hippocampus of the brain. I coined the term **immunoexcitotoxicity** to describe this process in the brain. This process also explains why infections are strongly linked to hepatic encephalopathy, because infections are highly inflammatory and activate brain microglia as well.

While most authorities attribute the problem to high levels of ammonium released from the intestines that are not metabolized by the damaged liver, there is some evidence that more is involved. For example, studies have shown that high levels of ammonia cause problems only if an infection is also present. High levels of ammonia alone had no effect.

As the encephalopathy worsens, especially if the person lapses into a coma, the arrival of death is close at hand. Earlier stages of encephalopathy can be reversed completely, especially the minimal stage.

The treatments listed below will also improve hepatic encephalopathy. In addition, L-carnitine has also been shown to dramatically improve this disorder. In one such study, researchers found that a dose of 2 grams of L-carnitine, taken twice a day, significantly lowered ammonia levels and improved the mental function of those taking the supplements.

Treatment for Cirrhosis

While there are no specific treatments for cirrhosis, there is a lot your doctor can do to manage it and try to prevent its progression.

Your outlook will depend on your overall health and whether you have developed any complications related to cirrhosis. This is true even when a person stops drinking.

First, if your cirrhosis is due to an underlying medical problem, such as nonalcoholic fatty liver disease, or chronic hepatitis B or C, or one of the rarer causes of cirrhosis, your doctor will treat those conditions.

If your cirrhosis is due to alcohol abuse, it is crucially important to get into an alcohol rehabilitation treatment program, because no progress in treating it can be made while a person is still drinking.

Diet

Alcoholic Cirrhosis

People with alcoholic cirrhosis should eat a balanced, healthy diet, containing mainly organic vegetables and organically raised meats, with a moderately reduced salt intake, and an emphasis on a higher intake of branched chain amino acids (valine, leucine, and isoleucine).

The branched chain amino acids have been shown to be beneficial in all types of cirrhosis, not just alcoholic forms. I once treated a man who had just undergone back surgery and his doctors could not get the wound to heal. He was known as a severe alcoholic. On examination, I could see that his back wound had not healed at all. Knowing of the beneficial effect in such cases of adding branched chain amino acids to his diet, I immediately started him on the amino acid combination. His wound healed completely within three weeks.

In all cases of alcoholic cirrhosis, all alcohol should be avoided, even wine.

Non-absorbable Disaccharides and Polyethylene Glycol

Lactulose, a sugar-like substance that is not absorbed, has been shown to improve hepatic encephalopathy in many studies, but not all. Polyethylene glycol seems to work faster in reversing symptoms than lactulose.

Antibiotics

Antibiotics that are not absorbed seem to work better than absorbable antibiotics. These antibiotics act on bacteria in the intestine and colon, which can be a major source of ammonia, as well as other toxic compounds. Careful studies have shown that using both of these, antibiotics and lactulose together, had the best results in reversing the damaging effects on the brain associated with cirrhosis.

Natural Products for Protecting and Treating Liver Diseases

Probiotics

Probiotics, especially when combined with prebiotics, appears to be effective in reducing hepatic encephalopathy. In one interesting study, 17 patients were given yogurt containing a mixture of probiotic organisms, and a control group of eight patients with cirrhosis and minimal hepatic encephalopathy were given yogurt without probiotics. Those given the probiotic yogurt demonstrated a significant improvement in a number of cognitive tests. The yogurt contained *Lactobacilus bulgaricus, Streptococcus thermophilius, L. acidophilus, L. casei,* and several strains of bifidobacteria. Interestingly, even though the patients eating the yogurt demonstrated significant improvements in mental function, there was no improvement in ammonia levels or inflammatory cytokines. All of the probiotic bacteria released lactose, which may have supplied fuel for the impaired brain cells.

Zinc

It is known that cirrhosis is associated with low blood and liver zinc levels. A review of four major trials containing a total of 247 cirrhotic patients demonstrated that, at least with mild cases of hepatic encephalopathy, zinc, when used along with lactulose, significantly improved the neuropsychiatric symptoms. A safe dose of zinc would be 50 mg of zinc picolinate daily.

Nano-Curcumin

Curcumin, a compound isolated from the spice turmeric, has a number of properties beneficial in treating liver disorders, especially fibrosis and cirrhosis. Of most importance is its antiviral properties, which have been shown to inhibit replications of the HIV virus, herpes simplex-1 virus, influenza virus, human papillomavirus, hepatitis B, and hepatitis C. Curcumin has been shown to also suppress the escape of these viruses by mutations.

Curcumin is also one of the more powerful anti-inflammatory products, reduces immune damage to the liver and other tissues, and most importantly is a powerful inhibitor of transforming growth factor Beta (TGF-ß1), a factor most involved in liver fibrosis and cirrhosis. Curcumin also enhances all the liver anti-oxidant enzymes, increases glutathione levels, and enhances the flow of bile from the liver.

Treatment with curcumin has been shown to dramatically improve alcoholic liver damage by reducing oxidative stress, inhibiting lipid peroxidation, reducing scar formation, and suppressing inflammatory cytokine release. By these same mechanisms, curcumin reduces the accumulation of fat in the liver, and is especially beneficial in treating NASH, the more inflammatory fatty liver disorder.

In one study examining 70 patients with cirrhosis, researchers found that those taking 1000 mg of curcumin a day demonstrated significant improvement in their quality-of-life measures, including mental health scores such as emotional function and depression, and showed physical improvements in such things as fatigue, vitality, itching, appetite, jaundice, interest in sex, joint pains, and physical functioning.

Curcumin has also been shown to reduce the toxicity of several drugs, such as acetaminophen.

Among all the flavonoids, curcumin has the most powerful anticancer effectiveness against a large number of cancer types, including hepatocellular cancer. In addition, curcumin enhances conventional chemotherapy treatments and protects normal tissue and organs against damage by these chemotherapy agents. It also improves radiation tumor-killing treatments and protects normal tissues against damage by the radiation.

Curcumin has a high margin of safety. As with many flavonoids, curcumin as a raw product is poorly absorbed. The Nano-Curcumin form is highly absorbable and distributed to all areas of the body, including the brain. And, unlike raw curcumin, it is water soluble.

How to take Nano-Curcumin. Nano-Curcumin, made by the One Planet Nutrition company, comes in a 250 mg capsule. The usual dose is one capsule, taken three times a day, 20 minutes before a meal. For treating a more advanced stage of the disease, one can take two to three capsules, three times a day, 20 minutes before a meal.

Because of its strong iron chelating properties, it would be best to take the Nano-Curcumin with your vitamin C supplement, as vitamin C prevents the iron chelation. Those with iron excess, as with hemochromatosis, should take the curcumin with meals, and vitamin C should be taken between meals.

Nano-Quercetin

As with curcumin, quercetin is poorly absorbed when taken orally. This problem has been overcome by nanosizing it, which means using a special process to reduce the size of the supplement particles into a below ultra-small size (nano). This not only increases absorption from the intestines and stomach, but also increases its distribution within cells and tissues.

Quercetin has powerful antioxidant, anti-inflammatory, anti-microbial, antifungal, antidiabetic, anticancer, and antiallergy properties. It has also been studied rather extensively in regard to cirrhosis and other liver disorders. In one such study, using a rat model of chemical-induced cirrhosis of an advanced degree, researchers found that quercetin, in a moderate dose, not only prevented much of the damage; it could also reverse a great deal of liver damage already caused by a powerful liver toxin (carbon tetrachloride).

They observed in these animals a chemical-caused cell death, fibrosis (scarring), infiltration of inflammatory cells, a high collagen content, extensive lipid peroxidation, and very high levels of nitric oxide (which enhances inflammation and cell damage). Quercetin given to the animals for 3 weeks greatly improved the histological picture of the liver, reduced the scarring, dramatically reduced the lipid peroxidation, and returned nitric oxide levels to normal.

All tissue and organ damage caused by inflammation involves high levels of nitric oxide (produced by inducible nitric oxide synthase—iNOS). Quercetin strongly reduces nitric oxide levels back to normal concentrations. With the fad of taking supplements to raise nitric oxide production in tissues, I fear an aggravation of such damage will be occurring more often. Nitric oxide is a two-edged sword—sometimes good and sometimes very harmful. This practice of increasing nitric oxide levels would be especially dangerous in people with liver disorders.

It is also important to note that very high doses of quercetin can actually be harmful (far beyond that recommended here). Only the moderate dose was effective and safe. Nano-Quercetin comes in a dose of 250 mg per capsule, which if taken three to four times a day would be adequate and safe. It should always be taken with food because it can lower blood sugar.

Quercetin has also been shown to be beneficial in cases of fatty liver disease, especially with the more serious nonalcoholic steatohepatitis (NASH), which is worse than the rather benign nonalcoholic fatty liver disease (NAFLD), in that NASH is accompanied by greater inflammation, high levels of free radicals and lipid peroxidation, and extensive scarring. NASH, if not corrected, can progress to full-blown cirrhosis and a higher risk of developing a hepatocellular carcinoma of the liver.

In one such study, researchers found that quercetin significantly inhibited fatty liver disease and protected against the development of the more serious disorder, NASH. One of the interesting findings was how the quercetin was inhibiting liver damage. Other studies suggested that the accumulation of fat in the liver was linked to abnormal microorganisms being present in the colon and intestines—the probiotics. It seems that these abnormal organisms generate ethanol-type alcohol, disrupt liver metabolism, and stimulate liver inflammation—a combination that is very harmful to the liver. The quercetin corrected the imbalance in colon probiotics, dramatically lowered the ethanol levels and lipid peroxidation, and prevented the oxidative stress that ultimately damaged the liver, causing fat to accumulate in the organ.

In addition, quercetin corrected the insulin sensitivity problem, which plays a major role in the development of fatty liver diseases. Another item of interest was that quercetin increased the concentration of a special bacteria called *Akkermansin muciniphila*, which is important in preventing obesity. Obesity plays a major role in fatty liver disease.

Quercetin powerfully inhibits liver inflammation and increases the production of short-chain fatty acids (SCFAs), which are critical for maintaining the health of the cells lining the intestine and preventing a leaky gut problem. One of these SCFAs, butyrate, is a powerful inhibitor of colon cancer.

Another relatively common cause of liver cirrhosis is biliary obstruction (cholestasis)—that is, obstruction of the bile ducts within the liver. This increases the level of certain inflammatory and toxic substances, leading to severe progressive damage to the liver and ultimately to cirrhosis.

Several studies have shown that quercetin can reverse much of the damage caused by bile duct obstruction. In one such study, using an animal model of the disorder, it was shown that quercetin reduced the pressure within the bile ducts, reduced fibrosis, and calmed the inflammatory reaction in the liver. The benefits were quite impressive. Other things have also shown benefits in biliary obstruction (cholestasis), such as S-adenosyl-L-methionine (SAMe) and N-acetyl-L-cysteine (NAC). In such liver diseases (cholestasis), we see very low levels of vitamin E and glutathione, which makes the liver highly susceptible to oxidative stress damage.

Another condition we see in cases of cirrhosis is damage to the lungs, the so-called **hepatopulmonary syndrome**. In this condition, the damaged liver floods the circulation with very high levels of nitric oxide, which damages the lungs by causing low oxygen levels and over-dilated blood vessels in the lungs (vasodilation). Quercetin was not only shown to improve the liver, but also to significantly reduce lung damage by lowering the extremely high nitric oxide levels back to normal and by reducing inflammation in the lungs.

Cirrhosis is also associated with kidney damage, the so-called **hepatorenal syndrome**. Quercetin also improves the kidneys and prevents further damage to them.

The bottom line is that quercetin, a safe compound, inhibits many of the processes that cause liver diseases and thereby protects the liver from harm.

How to take Nano-Quercetin. The most effective and safest dose of Nano-Quercetin is 250 mg taken three times a day with meals. For more severe liver disease, one can take two capsules three to four times a day with food.

Nano-Silymarin

One of the most studied natural compounds for liver disorders is silymarin, which is extracted from the milk thistle plant. As with the previous two natural compounds, silymarin is also poorly absorbed as the natural product. The Nano-Silymarin product is very well absorbed and penetrates the liver very effectively. Most studies have been done using the raw silymarin, but some other higher absorption products have shown better effects for liver protection and treatment of liver damage.

Most animal studies have been done using mice and rats. One study used baboons. In this study, researchers fed the baboons a meal containing high levels of ethanol-type alcohol for 36 months to produce liver cirrhosis. Half of the baboons were then given silymarin for 1 year and 18 months. Their liver was examined by liver biopsy every 6 months. The researchers also measured typical liver enzymes, as well as a powerful lipid peroxidation product called **4-hydroxynoneal** (4-HNE). The baboons given the alcohol develop extremely high levels of 4-HNE in their liver, as well as elevated liver enzymes and severe histological liver damage.

Those given the silymarin demonstrated a significantly improved histological picture on their biopsies and a dramatic lowering of the destructive compound 4-HNE. This is impressive as this lipid peroxidation product (4-HNE) is not neutralized by the usual vitamin antioxidants. While some earlier human studies either found moderate improvement in liver damage or no improvement, in most of these studies the poorly absorbed form of the silymarin was used in a low dose.

A recent review of silymarin used for liver diseases found that using clinical studies of people with both alcoholic and nonalcoholic liver diseases, silymarin significantly reduced deaths from cirrhosis. It was also beneficial in cases of drug-induced liver damage and diabetes-linked liver damage. The review led to the recommendations that treatment is most successful when started early in the course of the disease when the damage is less severe, and the regenerative capacity of the liver is still high. Silymarin has a high margin of safety and tolerability.

While silymarin is not considered a treatment for viral hepatitis itself, several studies have demonstrated improved quality-of-life measures, reduced jaundice, an improved histological picture, less fibrosis, and a reduction in bilirubin levels in those who took silymarin regularly.

How to take Nano-Silymarin. A safe and effective dose of Nano-Silymarin would be one to two capsules taken three to four times a day with food. It comes in 250 mg capsules.

DHA (Docosahexaenoic Acid)

Mice fed diets low in omega-3 fatty acids develop fatty livers and insulin resistance, just as we see in people. Studies have also shown that people who develop NAFLD consume a much lower ratio of omega-3 fatty acids to saturated fats, meaning they are deficient in omega-3 fats.

Studies of people having cirrhosis demonstrated that they had very low levels of one of the principal components of omega-3 fatty acids called DHA (docosahexaenoic acid) and that their level of DHA correlated with the progression of the disease, meaning that the worse their liver disease becomes, the lower the level of DHA in their liver. Other studies using animals have shown that DHA can significantly reduce the liver damage done by carbon tetrachloride, a powerful liver-destroying chemical.

Scarring of the liver, called *fibrosis*, causes most of the damage associated with cirrhosis. Interestingly, DHA powerfully inhibits the factor that causes most of the scarring called TGF-ß1, as well as other factors linked to liver scarring.

Inflammation is the main culprit in liver diseases, and an inflammatory cytokine called *tumor necrosis factor-alpha* (TNF-alpha) appears to be the main driver of liver inflammation. Studies have shown that omega-3 fatty acids powerfully suppress this inflammatory cytokine, as well as other inflammatory cytokines (IL-1ß, IL-6, and IFN-gamma).

In addition, DHA has powerful anti-inflammatory and anti-oxidant effects that suppress the very process that does most of the damage to the liver in cirrhosis: free radial damage and inflammation. A meta-analysis of nine clinical studies in which omega-3 oils were used to treat fatty liver disease demonstrated a significant reduction in elevated liver enzymes, and only minor benefits in reducing fibrosis. The problem with these studies is that they used a mixture of EPA and DHA and not pure DHA, the most beneficial component of omega-3 oils. In addition, they used doses that were far too low.

DHA should be used in a dose of 2000 mg a day. Certain brands of these oils contain some EPA, but usually no more than 170–200 mg of EPA should be used per day. The Pure Encapsulation company makes a product called **DHA Ultimate** that contains 790 mg of pure DHA and 188 mg of EPA. The dose is two capsules taken twice a day with a meal. As with all oils, it should be kept in the refrigerator.

Magnesium and Selenium

Magnesium is a potent inhibitor of inflammation, and low levels of magnesium are associated with the development of inflammation and insulin resistance. In one very large study involving

13,504 people, researchers found that higher magnesium intakes reduced the mortality associated with liver diseases, especially people with NASH or alcoholic liver disease.

Liver fibrosis (scarring) is the stage of liver diseases—in such disorders as NASH, alcoholic hepatitis, viral hepatitis, and chemical-induced hepatitis—that progresses to major liver destruction and cirrhosis. And fibrosis is associated with a combination of inflammation, oxidant stress, insulin resistance, obesity, metabolic syndrome, and type 2 diabetes. All of these are linked to low magnesium levels in the blood and liver tissues.

We see significantly low magnesium levels in alcoholic hepatitis, NAFLD, and NASH. A study of 4166 people found that the higher the magnesium intake, the lower the incidence of liver fibrosis, especially among males. Other studies have confirmed this finding.

In addition, magnesium has been shown to lower hs-CRP, a measure of inflammation in the body, in people with the metabolic syndrome. Other studies have shown that magnesium supplementation improves insulin sensitivity and type 2 diabetes.

One of the common forms of liver failure is related to abuse of alcohol over a long period. By a complex process, mainly involving alcohol-induced immune-triggered inflammation, alcohol slowly destroys the liver leading to a progressive destructive process that starts as a fatty liver and progresses to full-blown hepatitis, fibrosis, and ultimately cirrhosis.

A very interesting study examined the effect of supplementing rats subjected to alcoholic liver damage with either magnesium alone, selenium alone, or a combination of selenium plus magnesium. Giving magnesium alone partially alleviated the liver damage, but selenium alone was even more powerful in protecting the livers of these animals. To their surprise, a combination of selenium plus magnesium was no more effective than using selenium alone.

It is known that alcoholics have deficiencies in both selenium and magnesium and that these deficiencies worsen as the liver destruction progresses. Low magnesium has been shown to increase liver scarring. Supplementing with magnesium corrected the elevated liver enzymes (AST, ALT, and GGT) and restored critical levels of antioxidants in the liver, such as glutathione-S-transferase, superoxide dismutase (SOD), and vitamin C.

Selenium plays an important role in building a very critical antioxidant enzyme called *glutathione peroxidase.* Deficiencies in selenium are associated with heart failure, increased cancer risk, and disorders of the liver, kidneys, and bones. The antioxidant enzyme SOD is critical because even when an alcoholic is abstaining from drinking, the free radical called *superoxide* is elevated, which is neutralized by the SOD enzyme.

The magnesium may have had less effectiveness than the selenium because too low a dose of magnesium was used. Higher doses have better effectiveness. Combining selenium with magnesium in this study did improve glutathione function significantly compared to when selenium or magnesium was used alone.

Selenium should never be taken in doses higher than 200 mcg a day. One can take 200 mcg daily for 2 weeks and then cut the dose to 100 mcg daily thereafter.

Alcohol abuse is also associated with deficiencies in vitamin E, vitamin C, zinc, copper, and carotenoids.

How to take selenium and magnesium. There are many formulations of magnesium—powder, capsules, and slow-release caplets. The powder can be dissolved in water, but taking it on an empty stomach can result in intestinal cramping and diarrhea. It is best taken with a meal. The dose is one scoop dissolved in a glass of water once or twice a day. The powdered form is made by the **Pure Encapsulation** company and includes a scoop that is measured to provide 250 mg of magnesium.

The time-release form of magnesium malate is probably the most tolerated form. This is made by www.jigsawhealth.com. The dose is two tablets, twice a day, taken with food.

The best form of selenium is selenomethionine in a dose of 100 mcg per capsule. Take one capsule with or without food per day.

Baicalin

Baicalin and baicalein are powerful compounds isolated from the plant **Scutellaria baicalensis**, also called *skullcap*. Baicalin, the most common form found after ingesting the product orally, has been shown to be anti-inflammatory, antioxidant, anti-angiogenesis, immune-regulatory, anti-obesity, antiviral, and anti-dyslipidemic. The skullcap plant has been used safely as a medicinal herb for thousands of years in Asia.

Following ingestion, the highest levels of baicalin are found in the liver and kidneys. Once in the bloodstream, baicalin easily passes through the blood brain barrier into the brain and spinal cord. Unfortunately, baicalin is poorly absorbed and does not dissolve in either water or oils. Special high-absorption forms have been shown to dramatically increase its benefits. Hopefully, we will soon have a Nano-Baicalin form, which would be highly absorbable.

Baicalin has very powerful antiviral properties, such as against the influenza virus, hepatitis B virus, cytomegalovirus, enteroviruses, coxsackie B virus, HIV virus, and herpes simplex viruses. Recent studies have also shown that combining baicalin with antiviral drugs, such as entecavir, greatly enhance the effectiveness of traditional treatments for hepatitis B.

Baicalin is also a major weapon against fatty liver diseases, such as NAFLD and NASH, based on its ability to enhance lipid metabolism and suppress generation of lipids within the liver. Baicalin enhances the entry of fats into the mitochondria, the principal site of their metabolism.

Baicalin has been shown to lower blood levels of triglycerides, total cholesterol, lower LDL, raise HDL, and lower abnormally elevated liver enzymes, such as AST and ALT. The higher doses of baicalin were shown to dramatically reverse fat-induced steatohepatitis (NASH). In addition, this compound suppresses liver fibrosis, oxidative stress, and systemic inflammation. Careful studies have shown that baicalin inhibits the cell-signaling compound called **TGF-ß1**, as well as other collagen-producing processes—that is, it suppresses scar formation in the liver.

As we saw with Nano-Curcumin, baicalin also enhances the levels of glutathione and superoxide dismutase (SOD) in the liver—two very important antioxidants. A recent study found that combining baicalin and curcumin significantly enhanced antioxidant protection of the liver by raising the level of two very important antioxidant cellular mechanisms: NrF2 and heme oxygenase-1.

Studies have shown that this interesting compound also reduces immune over-reactivity, a major process in all liver diseases. Several studies have demonstrated that baicalin reduces glucose intolerance, lowers abnormally high blood glucose, and reduces insulin resistance, which is involved in type 2 diabetes.

Another very useful property of baicalin is its ability to suppress liver damage caused by environmental toxins. For example, baicalin significantly reduces the liver and kidney damage caused by the painkiller acetaminophen. It has also been found to reduce liver inflammation caused by immune overstimulation, prevent damage by iron overload (as seen with hemochromatosis), and protect the liver against some very powerful chemical liver toxins.

Recent studies have also shown this compound to be effective in treating cholestatic liver injury, at least in experimental animals. One disease associated with cholestasis is **primary sclerosing cholangitis**, which normally affects young and middle-aged men. It is an autoimmune disorder that attacks bile ducts within the liver, impeding the flow of bile (cholestasis) and leading to intense scarring.

As we have seen, most liver disorders, no matter what the cause, have as their central pathological process immune-induced inflammation. Baicalin suppresses the powerful proinflammatory cytokines—TNF-alpha, IL-1ß, and IL-6—as well as the main cell triggers for inflammation NF_kB and NLRP3. This makes it a very powerful weapon against all liver diseases, including viral hepatitis.

Baicalin recently has been shown to be effective in treating minimal hepatic encephalopathy by its effects on protective brain mechanisms. Of real interest is the ability of baicalin to significantly reduce anxiety and depression.

Baicalin is a powerful weapon against hepatocellular carcinoma (primary liver cancer) by a number of processes. This cancer always develops from advanced stages of liver diseases associated with intense liver scarring and chronic inflammation of the liver. The powerful anti-inflammatory and antioxidant effects of this compound strikes at the very cause of liver cancer, thus preventing it from ever developing.

Baicalin can be purchased as a fine powder from a company called **Lift Mode**, which makes a number of natural plant extract powders. The cannister of powder comes with a small plastic spoon for measuring. The dose is one to two level spoonfuls twice to three times a day with meals. Baicalin can induce hypoglycemia, so it should be taken with meals. I suspend the powder in water and drink it before it can settle. I would switch to the Nano-Baicalin as soon as it is available.

Apigenin

Another plant extract that reduces liver fibrosis is apigenin, a flavonoid found in higher concentrations in celery, parsley, thyme, chamomile, and onions. A very recent study using mice exposed to a powerful liver-destroying chemical and another model of cholestasis found that, in both conditions, apigenin decreased the elevation of liver enzymes, signifying a reduction in injury to liver cells. It also suppressed the buildup of scar tissue (fibrosis) and lowered the concentration of TGF-ß1, the factor that is most responsible for liver fibrosis.

Apigenin is known for repairing the intestines and reducing inflammation of the lining of the intestines. Keep in mind that in most liver diseases we see a breakdown of the intestinal lining (leaky gut syndrome) allowing food particles and bacteria to enter the blood vessels supplying the liver. This can trigger intense inflammation in the liver.

Studies have also shown apigenin to be antidiabetic and an anti-obesity compound. Apigenin has been shown to activate genes that help burn fats, lower inflammatory cytokines, decrease insulin resistance, and markedly reduce total cholesterol levels as well as apolipoprotein B levels. These properties not only reduce liver disease and damage but also reduce the risk of atherosclerosis.

When nanoparticulate apigenin was tested against hepatocellular carcinoma, researchers found a significant slowing of the growth and spread of the cancer. The dose is two 50 mg capsules three times a day with meals.

Other Natural Compounds of Benefit

Luteolin, a compound found in higher levels in celery and artichokes, has shown some rather remarkable beneficial effects in cases of alcoholic liver damage and cases of chemical liver damage. A study in which mice were exposed to chronic binge alcohol feeding, found that luteolin, especially in higher doses, could relieve alcohol-induced fatty liver disease and prevent further progression to cirrhosis. One of the major effects of the luteolin was that it increased the level of special fibrosis (scar) dissolving enzymes (MMPs). Animal studies have shown that luteolin could completely reverse liver fibrosis. It also reduced liver fat accumulation and hepatocyte cell damage. Luteolin can be found in a dose of 100 mg per capsule. A safe dose would be two capsules taken three times a day with meals.

Pterostilbene has also been shown to reduce fat accumulation in the liver and to correct insulin resistance. Once absorbed, pterostilbene is converted in the tissues into resveratrol. The advantage is that pterostilbene is far better absorbed than resveratrol. Resveratrol has about 20% absorption from the gut, and pterostilbene has an 80% absorption rate. Insulin resistance can lead to type 2 diabetes, which is strongly associated with fatty liver disease. The dose of pterostilbene is 100 to 200 mg taken three times a day. It comes in 100 mg capsules.

Long-term consumption of whole broccoli in one study was found to significantly protect against the development of fatty liver diseases.

Hesperidin, another flavonoid found mostly in fruits, has been shown to be especially protective against iron toxicity in the liver and kidneys, as one would see in cases of hemochromatosis and other iron excess diseases. Hesperidin is very safe and is also associated with superior ability to strengthen veins. The dose is one 500 mg capsule taken three times a day with meals.

Vitamin C (buffered), B-complex vitamins (from Thorne Research or Pure Encapsulation), and vitamins K_2 and K_3 supply the liver with essential nutrients and have anti-inflammatory effects. Vitamin D_3 is essential for immune modulation and as an anti-inflammatory. The dose is 5000 IU a day. A serum vitamin D_3 level test should be done 3 weeks after starting therapy. The normal level is between 65 ng/ml and 100 ng/ml. Vitamin E, as a mixed tocopherol, should be taken in a dose of 400 IU a day. Mixed tocotrienols should be taken in a dose of 50 mg twice a day.

Finally, a study of cases associated with cirrhosis found that there was an inverse association with coffee drinking and mortality from cirrhosis. That is, the more coffee participants drank, the greater the reduction in dying from their disease. Coffee contains a number of antioxidants and flavonoids associated with reducing inflammation and oxidative stress.

L-carnitine has been shown to prevent muscle loss in cases of liver cirrhosis. The dose would be 1000 mg taken three times a day 30 minutes before a meal.

CHAPTER 15

Leaky Gut Syndrome and SIBO

The colon is the longest part of the intestines, and is the final part of the digestive system. Its function is to reabsorb fluids and process waste products from the body and prepare for their elimination.

One of the newer scientific discoveries is a link between the gut (stomach, small intestine, and colon) and the liver—the so-called gut-liver axis—which refers to the relationship between the gut, its microbiota (bacterial environment), and the liver.

That there is a flow between the gut and the liver makes sense because substances absorbed from the intestine travel by the portal blood vessels directly to the liver. This includes not only digested foods and drinks, but also various toxic substances released from the gut. Strongly linked to this gut-liver axis is the concept of a leaky gut (leaky gut syndrome) and an overgrowth of bacteria in the small intestine (SIBO).

The colon contains more cells in terms of microorganisms than there are cells within the human body. These microorganisms include some 100 trillion microorganisms of 200 species of bacteria, most of which are anaerobic forms. In addition, the colon contains viruses and fungi. At birth, the gut is sterile, and during the baby's travel along the mother's birth canal, the baby begins to acquire its first exposure to these microorganisms. Breast milk, and later solid foods following birth, then become the main source of these essential microorganisms.

The composition of these microorganisms is unique for each person and is maintained throughout life, except in cases where outside factors alter their composition, such as exposure to antibiotics, chemotherapy agents, stress, diet, aging, and various comorbid conditions. We call this unique pattern of bacteria our "microbial fingerprint." Another factor playing a role in the composition of these gut microbiota is the immune system. There is a two-way communication between the immune system and these gut organisms. The immune system helps shape the composition of our microbiota, and the gut microbiota modulates the immune system. You will recall, approximately 80% of the immune system is located within the walls of the gut.

Extensive studies have shown that there is a critical role played by the gut microbiota in a number of diseases, such as type 1 and 2 diabetes, obesity, cardiovascular diseases, metabolic disorders, and chronic liver diseases.

Normally, the cells lining the gut are positioned to be very close together (called *tight junctions*), to prevent purely digested substances and bacteria within the gut from ending up in the bloodstream, where they can cause immune reactions or direct toxic effects. In leaky gut syndrome, breaks occur in these intestinal tight junctions, allowing incompletely digested particles of food and bacteria to enter the bloodstream. Within the bloodstream, these unwelcome visitors are attacked by the immune system. In addition, these microorganisms are also carried directly to the liver where they can react with the liver's innate immune system—which includes what are called *Kupffer cells* and *stellate cells*.

When these liver immune cells are chronically activated, they can secrete inflammatory cytokines and other substances that can damage liver cells (hepatocytes).

Normally, the small intestine contains very few if any bacteria. In the condition called *small intestinal bacterial overgrowth* (SIBO), a large number of microorganisms begin to inhabit the small intestine. Diagnosis is based on finding more than 10^5 CFU (colony forming units)/ml from an aspiration sample of the duodenum. The most common symptoms of SIBO include bloating, abdominal discomfort, watery diarrhea, dyspepsia, weight loss, macrocytic anemia, and eventually hepatic steatosis (fatty liver).

Several conditions are associated with an increased incidence of SIBO. These include obesity, use of stomach acid–reducing medications, irritable bowel syndrome, low pancreatic enzyme production, and low ileocecal valve function. Gastric acid–reducing medications are a major cause of SIBO. Stomach acid kills most bacteria and other microorganisms swallowed during eating. Food is a major source of intestinal microorganisms. In fact, a recent study found that proton-pump inhibitors caused SIBO twice as often as irritable bowel syndrome, considered to be a major link to the condition.

In one study of 38 patients with nonalcoholic fatty liver disease (NAFLD), researchers found a 39% incidence of SIBO. There is some evidence that SIBO plays an important role in NAFLD, which is increasing dramatically worldwide.

Abnormal gut permeability is also increasing dramatically. SIBO is also common in cases of liver cirrhosis.

In my opinion, two drugs are the main cause for the dramatic increase in NAFLD caused by SIBO and a leaky gut: gastric acid–reducing medications and nonsteroidal anti-inflammatory medications (NSAIDS), which are both widely used. NSAIDS are known to cause disruption of the intestinal tight junctions, leading to a leaky gut. Leaky gut can also follow bouts of gastroenteritis. Both chemotherapy and radiation in the area of the intestines during cancer treatments can also result in a leaky gut problem. SIBO is also much more common in the elderly than younger individuals.

When combined with a leaky gut problem, these microorganisms flood into the liver's portal blood supply and end up within the liver itself. Once in the liver, these bacterial substances react with liver-based immune cells through special receptors (toll-like receptors), which activate intense immune reactions. As long as the small intestine is overgrown with these organisms, the liver will be exposed to continuous immune reactions that will in turn generate high levels of inflammatory cytokines, resulting in chronic liver inflammation. Inflammation is always accompanied by generation of high levels of free radicals and lipid peroxidation products, both of which can cause extensive liver damage. Over time, this constant inflammation will lead to fibrosis of the liver, a condition we call cirrhosis. In some instances, inflammatory cirrhosis can lead to liver cancer (hepatocarcinoma).

SIBO also plays a major role in nonalcoholic steatohepatitis (NASH), a condition more likely to progress into hepatocarcinoma and/or liver failure. Certain bacteria release high levels of lipopolysaccharide, a powerful immune stimulant, which when entering the liver can cause severe inflammation and liver damage. Other substances released by bacteria in the intestine include lipopeptides, unmethylated DNA, and double-stranded RNA, all of which can induce inflammation and high levels of free radicals in the liver.

SIBO plays a role in other liver disorders, such as alcoholic cirrhosis, liver fibrosis, and viral hepatitis. The liver also plays a role in microbiota composition, and ultimately SIBO by its regulation of bile acid release into the gut. Bile acids have a bacterial suppressing effect, thus controlling gut microbiota profiles. With liver diseases, we see a reduction in the release of bile acids by the gall bladder into the intestines, and this allows the gut bacteria to overgrow—thus leading to SIBO. As the severity of the liver disease advances, so does the prevalence of SIBO.

Obesity plays a major role in progression of liver disease for a number of reasons. SIBO is more common in obese individuals and obesity is associated with high levels of inflammation, which also leads to fatty liver disease and steatohepatitis. This also means that obesity is strongly associated with liver cancer. There is substantial evidence that obesity is a more powerful contributor of liver disease than are hepatitis viruses.

You learned earlier that insulin resistance plays a major role in fatty liver disease. In conjunction with insulin resistance is the contribution played by translocated bacteria from the gut—that is, bacteria that leak out of the gut and head for the liver.

Insulin resistance, like translocated gut microbiota, drive intense inflammation—that is, they are working together to cause havoc within the liver. Bile acids also help protect the gut barrier, so as to prevent microorganism translocation to the liver. As the liver damage progresses, it produces less bile acids and, as a result, the likelihood of a leaky gut increases. You can now see how the interplay between the liver and the gut can drive liver diseases.

Fortunately, this also gives us a number of weapons to combat liver disease. The most important of these is the use of probiotics, prebiotics, and synbiotics. For example, it has been shown that *Lactobacillus*, *Bifidobacteria*, and *Satreptococcus* strains of bacteria can inhibit the growth of certain Gram-negative pathogenic (disease causing) bacteria.

In another study, researchers found that *Lactobacillus casei* strain Shirota (Lcs) could dramatically improve the symptoms of NASH, including significant improvement in the histological damage to the liver. In addition, this probiotic reduced serum tri-glycerides and total cholesterol levels. Importantly, this specific probiotic also significantly improved insulin resistance.

Fructose is a major cause for dietary-induced fatty liver disease and insulin resistance. One study found that *Lactobacillus casei* Shirota could protect fructose-fed mice from developing liver steatosis (fatty liver).

Lactobacillus paracasei was found in one study to lower the level of inflammatory cytokines in NASH patients, which you will recall is the driving force behind the liver damage. Using a NAFLD model, researchers also found that *Lactobacillus plantarum* MA2 and *Lactobacillus* A7 were effective in lowering serum lipids.

Another strain of *Lactobacillus plantarum* (N116) was shown to improve liver function and decrease fat accumulation in the livers of diet-induced fatty liver disease in rats.

Lactobacillus rhamnosus, given to animal models of NAFLD, was shown to increase the number of beneficial bacteria in the colon, improve gut barrier function, and reduce the level of inflammation. Another strain of bifidobacteria was shown to improve visceral fat accumulation and thus improve insulin sensitivity in a model of metabolic syndrome.

One research group found that bifidobacterial species were more effective in reducing hepatic fat accumulation than were the *lactobacillus* species.

Prebiotics were also found to be effective. In one such prebiotic study, researchers demonstrated a reduction in inflammatory cytokine levels and improved intestinal permeability in mice.

While most of these studies utilized a single bacterium, other studies found that utilizing a mixture of probiotic organisms was significantly more effective. One such mixture, called VSL#3, which contained *Bifidobacteria breve, B. longum, B. infantis, Streptococcus thermophilus, L. plantarum, L. acidophilus,*

L. paracasei, and *L. delbrueckii-subspecies bulgarisus,* was shown to reduce fat accumulation in the liver, lower elevated liver enzymes, and improve insulin sensitivity in a model of NAFLD.

In another study, researchers found that a combination of *B. infantis, L acidophilus,* and *Bacillus cereus* improved gut dysbiosis and liver function by suppressing immune receptors in liver cells.

Clinical studies have confirmed what was found in animals given these probiotic combinations. In one randomized clinical study, in which researchers used the VSL#3 probiotic combination mentioned earlier on obese children with biopsy proven nonalcoholic steatohepatitis (NAFLD) for 4 months, found significant improvement in their liver function.

Similar excellent results were seen using a combination of *L. rhamnosus GG, L. bulgaricus,* and *Streptococcus thermophilus* in adults with NAFLD.

Others found impressive improvement in insulin sensitivity and inflammation in cases of NAFLD when these probiotics were used.

As in the animal studies using probiotics, prebiotics were also beneficial in fatty liver diseases. For example, researchers found that adding the inulin-type fructans prebiotic to the diet of NASH patients in a double-blind study, decreased the ALT and AST liver enzymes significantly. In one study, combining prebiotics (oligofructose and inulin—50:50) increased the growth of *Bifidobacterial* and *Faecalibacterium prausnitzii,* two probiotics associated with lowering serum levels of lipopolysacchride, the powerful stimulator of inflammatory cytokines released from the gut.

The use of mixtures of probiotic species, usually with prebiotic fibers (called *synbiotics*), has been shown to improve levels of fasting blood sugar, triglycerides, and inflammatory cytokines both in obese and lean patients with NAFLD.

Another impressive method of both correcting leaky gut problems and regulating liver metabolism is use of N-butyrate, a short-chain fatty acid. Butyrate has been shown to be a major fuel for endothelial cells lining the GI tract. In one study, researchers found that a combination of a probiotic and N-butyrate modulated liver energy metabolism (lipogenesis and gluconeogenesis), improved regulation of fat entry into adipocytes (fat cells), corrected intestinal permeability, and altered appetite regulation by the brain.

Certain plant extracts can also play a role in correcting fatty liver problems through regulation of microbiota in the gut. For example, berberine has potent antibacterial properties and significantly improves blood sugar control in diabetics.

Studies have also demonstrated the ability of berberine to improve steatohepatitis and to lower body weight, serum lipids, glucose, insulin levels, and inflammatory cytokines in experimental animal models of NASH.

Resveratrol has been shown to prevent obesity and NASH by regulating gut microbiota. Because of pterostilbene's superior absorption, and that once absorbed it is transformed into resveratrol, this product may be a better choice to control both obesity and fatty liver disease.

One's diet also regulates gut microbiota composition. For example, the typical Western diet promotes pro-inflammatory-type microbiota such as *Bacteroides*, whereas the Mediterranean diet promotes the growth of anti-inflammatory microbiota such as *Bifidobacteria* species or *Akkerrnasia*, both of which promote immune tolerance to foods and strengthens the intestinal barrier tight junctions.

Excess alcohol consumption also increases the risk of leaky gut–based liver damage by breaking down the gut's tight junction intestinal barrier. Alcoholics experience increased liver damage based both on direct toxicity of alcohol on liver cells and an exposure to high levels of toxins and bacterial products from the leaky gut, the so-called endotoxin (autotoxic) effect. In fact, several studies have shown that susceptibility to liver cirrhosis depends heavily on the composition of the gut microbiota.

This link to gut bacterial composition was clearly demonstrated using germ-free animal models in which the animals having no microorganisms in their colon were used. When microbiota from alcoholic patients with liver disease were transplanted into the colon of these germ-free animals and then exposed to alcohol, a high percentage developed cirrhosis and leaky gut, whereas the germ-free animals having microbiota from alcoholic patients without liver disease, had a much lower incidence of liver damage.

It was also demonstrated that once the liver damage was established in the animals, transplanting the microbiota from alcoholic patients without liver damage actually improved the pathological damage in the mice. This shows that liver damage from alcohol is dependent on the person's composition of microorganisms within their colon. Anti-inflammatory species, such as *Bifidobacteria* and *Lactobacillus*, were protective against alcohol-induced liver damage.

Other studies have shown that these two bacterial species can improve liver function tests, strengthen gut barriers, reduce levels of pro-inflammatory cytokines and bacterial endotoxins in the blood, and stimulate histological improvement in cases of liver steatosis and liver inflammation.

The probiotic composition within the colon can also have an effect on the risk of SIBO. Cancer patients frequently develop SIBO secondary to the treatments. One study found that treating SIBO in cancer patients with a mix of *Bifidobacteria* species could significantly reduce SIBO in these patients.

One of the great fears associated with NAFLD and NASH is the eventual development of liver cancer—hepatocellular carcinoma. Examinations of patients with this cancer have shown that they have a particular mix of colon microbiota, which include *Bacteroides*, *Ruminococcus*, *Enterococcus*, and decreased levels of the *Bifidobacteria* and *Blautia* species when compared to cirrhotics without liver cancer. Other studies have shown that certain probiotic mixtures, such as *L rhamnosus* GG, viable *E Coli Nissle* 1917 (EcN), and heat-inactivated VSL## caused a significant reduction in the growth of this type of liver cancer, and that reducing the circulating level of lipopolysaccharide (LPS) using antibiotics (which kill pathogenic bacteria) prevented the growth of liver cancer.

Particular strains of *Bifidobacteria*, *Lactobacillus* and *E. Coli*, *Propionibacterium*, *Bacillus*, and *Sacchraomyces* have a beneficial effect on immune receptors, cell-death caspases, and inflammatory cytokines that in total reduce inflammation in the liver.

Conclusions

Bacterial overgrowth in the small intestine (SIBO), which normally has very few if any bacteria, is strongly linked to the leaky gut syndrome, where the normal tight junction intestinal barriers are defective. This allows bacteria, fungi, fragments of microorganisms, and bacterial toxins (endotoxins) to enter the portal blood vessels where they can trigger immune reactions directly in the blood. Upon entering the liver, these same products can further activate special immune cells in the liver called Kupffer cells and stellate cells. Upon activation, these cells release a number of inflammatory products, such as cytokines and chemokines, which cause variable degrees of damage to liver structures.

This chronic inflammation causes fat to accumulate in liver cells, a condition called steatosis—or nonalcoholic fatty liver disease (NAFLD). As the condition accelerates, producing higher levels of inflammation and liver destruction, we see the appearance of increasing levels of liver damage. The accumulation of fat in the liver cells alters liver metabolism and can further increase liver inflammation. Over time, a process of fibrosis develops, which can further damage the liver's structure—a condition we call nonalcoholic steatohepatitis (NASH). In some individuals, chronic inflammation in the liver will lead to the development of liver cell cancer—hepatocellular carcinoma.

As you have seen, the particular composition of the microbiota within the colon plays a major role in one's susceptibility to liver damage, as well as the conditions leading up to this damage, such as insulin resistance, increased intestinal permeability, SIBO, and ultimately, levels of inflammation.

Importantly, it has been demonstrated that one can prevent and even treat these conditions by using a mixture of special probiotics, prebiotics, and other nutritional products. Diet, exercise, and stress reduction all play a role in preventing these conditions. The easiest way to take advantage of these methods is to buy a probiotic that contains at least four or five strains of *Bifidobacteria* and five species of *Lactobacillus* containing at least 20 billion CFU. These probiotics should be taken at least once a week. In addition, adding prebiotics, which are the foods for the bacteria, will further enhance the beneficial effects by stimulating the growth of species not available in commercial products, as well as feed the probiotics in your supplement. The two best prebiotics include inulins and galacto-oligosaccharides (GOS). These can be taken daily, or at least three times a week, preferably between meals or at bedtime.

CHAPTER 16

Liver Tumors

The largest number of deaths from liver cancer occurs in third-world countries and specific locations in the Western world. Worldwide, hepatocellular carcinoma, the leading cause of primary liver cancer, is the second-leading cause of cancer deaths.

In the U.S., like elsewhere, liver cancer is a rare cancer, but people do die from it here. This is unfortunate, as most of these cancers could be avoided, in my opinion.

Primary liver cancer is not a serious risk unless one suffers from a chronic liver condition, such as a viral hepatitis, has a fatty liver disease, has cirrhosis from any cause, has advanced fibrosis of the liver, abuses alcohol, smokes, is exposed chronically to a known liver toxin, or has diabetes. In rare instances, a genetic abnormality puts one in a higher risk category, mainly making the person more susceptible to liver damage by one of the conditions listed previously.

What Is Liver Cancer?

Like other types of cancer, liver cancer is a disease caused by an uncontrolled division of abnormal cells in a part of the body.

Normally, cells in the body will grow and divide to replace old or damaged cells. This growth is highly regulated, and once enough cells are produced to replace the old ones, normal cells will stop dividing. Cancer occurs when there is an error in this regulation and cells continue to reproduce uncontrolled.

Because cancers behave so much like the normal healing process, cancer is sometimes characterized as a wound that never heals. When we have an injury, numerous cell mechanisms are activated to repair the damage, including generations of new cells from stem cells. Normally, when the healing is complete, the process is shut off and the cells stop reproducing so fast. In cancer, for a number of reasons, this process of cell proliferation doesn't stop. Unlike normal cells, the cancer cells become immortal.

Considerable evidence suggests that the driving force for this uncontrolled cell generation is chronic, low-grade inflammation. We see cancers developing in tissues and organs that are constantly inflamed by many different processes, such as an injury, an infection, a parasite infection, an autoimmune disorder, or exposure to a chemical agent.

There are as many types of cancer as there are types of tissues. Liver cancer begins in the cells of the liver. There are several different types of liver cancer. The most common type of liver cancer is hepatocellular carcinoma, which begins in the main type of liver cell (hepatocyte). Other types of liver cancer, such as intrahepatic cholangiocarcinoma, cancers of the extrahepatic bile ducts, cancer involving the ampulla of Vater (a small opening in the small intestine), and hepatoblastoma, are much less common.

Cancer originating at other sites, such as colon cancer or breast cancer, which metastasize to the liver are more common than cancer that begins primarily in the liver cells. These cancers that metastasize, or spread, to the liver are called *metastatic cancer* rather than *liver cancer*. This type of spreading cancer is named after the organ in which it began—such as metastatic colon cancer to describe cancer that begins in the colon and spreads to the liver.

Cancer that begins in the liver is called *primary liver cancer*. Metastatic cancer, which spreads to the liver from another organ, such as the pancreas or colon, is known as a secondary cancer.

Who Gets Liver Cancer?

As stated, this rather rare cancer is most often associated with preexisting liver disease. About 42,230 people are diagnosed with liver cancer each year in the U.S., with about 30,000 deaths resulting from this disease every year. This nasty cancer does not respond well to any conventual treatment. It is estimated that 30,230 deaths (20,300 men and 9,930 women) from this disease will occur each year, according to Cancer.net. The incidence of liver cancer has tripled in the U.S. since 1980, and is increasing rapidly.

Men are about 70% more likely to develop liver cancer than are women, making it the fifth most common cause of cancer death in men. Researchers have discovered that a hormone secreted by fat cells, that is present at higher levels in women, can reduce the risk of liver cells from becoming cancerous. Asian Americans and Pacific Islanders have the highest rates of liver cancer in the U.S.

In the United States, Japan, and several Western countries, hepatocellular carcinoma is most often associated with a chronic hepatitis C infection. Approximately 30 to 50% of cases fall into this category. (Approximately 85% of hepatitis C infections become chronic.) Another 10 to 20% are related to alcohol abuse, and hepatitis B accounts for 10 to 15% of cases. What is called **cryptogenic cirrhosis**—that is, cirrhosis for which a cause is not known—accounts for 15% to as high as 50% of cases of this cancer. Further examination of these cases usually discloses a cause. Genetic disorders, such as Wilson's disease, alpha1-antitrypsin deficiency, and hemochromatosis accounts for a minor number of cases.

In sub-Saharan Africa and Asia, hepatitis B is the leading cause of this cancer. Exposure to foods contaminated with aflatoxin, a fungal mycotoxin found in cereals and peanuts, is also a leading cause of this cancer in Northern Africa and Asia. Aflatoxins are found even in most expensive brands of peanut butter in the U.S.

The highest risk of liver cancer is in people having more than one infection (hepatitis B, hepatitis delta virus, or HIV infection), diabetics, smokers, older individuals, those who drink alcohol (especially to excess), people having advanced stages of liver fibrosis or cirrhosis from any cause, and those who use a liver toxic artificial sweetener or excitotoxic food additive (MSG, hydrolyzed protein, soy protein extract, or isolate, etc.).

Liver Cancer, Obesity, and Metabolic Disorders

There is also a strong link to being overweight and especially being obese. One study found that overweight individuals had a 17% higher risk of developing the cancer than individuals of normal weight, and that obese individuals had an 89% higher risk. In fact, a study of 900,000 people followed for 16 years found a strong link between obesity and many types of cancer, including liver cancer. Another study found that obesity increased the risk of a person with cryptogenic cirrhosis developing a liver cancer by threefold. The same study found that alcohol drinking increased the risk of developing this cancer by 11-fold. Even more evidence comes from a study of a very large number of American adults that found that the risk of dying from liver cancer was 4.5-fold higher in obese men as compared to men of normal weight.

Patients with either hepatitis C or B who are obese are at a much higher risk of liver cancer than normal-weight individuals. While no studies have been done, I would suspect that obese people using aspartame, Splenda (sucralose), or excitotoxin food additives would also be at a much greater risk for liver cancer.

Studies have also shown that having type 2 diabetes puts a person at a much higher risk for liver cancer. For example, one study found a 7.5-fold increased risk should a person exhibit insulin resistance, the cause for type 2 diabetes. Interestingly, being obese and having diabetes together is much worse. One such study found a 100-fold increase in liver cancer when the two conditions were both present in the same person. A study from Sweden found that having diabetes increased a person's risk of developing a liver cancer by 4.5-fold, should other risk factors coexist. Having diabetes alone still increased the risk by threefold.

Fructose, especially in the form of high-fructose corn syrup, significantly increases liver cancer risk. Remember, fructose consumption was strongly associated with fatty liver diseases. A European study found that nonalcoholic fatty liver disease (NAFLD) was found in 74% of obese patients and 25% of those with nonalcoholic steatohepatitis (NASH). It was also discovered that 40 to 70% of people with type 2 diabetes also have NAFLD.

Fatty Liver Disease and the Risk of Liver Cancer

NAFLD, a condition of simple fatty liver without inflammation, is rarely associated with liver cancer, but it does happen. People with NASH, which is more advanced than NAFLD and much more inflammatory, have a significantly higher risk of developing liver cancer. Again, having any other condition known to worsen liver damage, such as obesity, type 2 diabetes, exposure to liver toxic substances, having a chronic viral hepatitis infection, smoking, drinking alcohol, and being older would put these people at a much higher risk than simple NAFLD alone.

Approximately 25 to 30% of the American population has a fatty liver and 25% of these individuals will advance to NASH. Of the NASH patients, 25% will eventually develop cirrhosis, which will put them in a high-risk category of developing liver cancer. Interestingly, while most NAFLD is rather benign, cirrhosis is twice as likely to develop with this disorder than with chronic hepatitis C, mainly because it is far more common. In fact, cirrhosis associated with NAFLD is rapidly becoming the leading cause for liver transplants. Hepatitis C–caused cirrhosis is actually declining as a cause.

The presence of a fatty liver with inflammation (NASH) increases the risk of developing liver cancer in those infected chronically with the hepatitis C virus by two- to threefold. Interestingly, having a fatty liver and hepatitis B infection actually lowers one's risk of liver cancer. This is because the fat in this condition reduced the number of viruses in the liver.

Patients with NAFLD and liver cancer are usually older, female, and have several metabolic disorders, such as type 2 diabetes, insulin resistance, or metabolic syndrome. Unfortunately, their liver cancer has the same extremely low survival rate as that found in men.

Alcoholic Liver Disease and Liver Cancer

Alcohol abuse is a major cause for liver cirrhosis in most countries, and cirrhosis is powerfully linked to the risk of developing liver cancer. One large study of almost 10,000 people found a linear relationship between the amount of alcohol consumed daily and the risk of developing liver cancer. Moderate drinkers (less than three drinks a day) had no significant increased risk, but three drinks or more substantially raised risk. At 50 grams of drink a day to 100 grams a day, the risk leaped from 29 to 66%, respectively. More than three drinks a day further increased the risk.

The authors of this study recognized that it was very difficult to evaluate all the factors involved, such as silent viral infections, diets, genetics, exposure to other liver toxins, use of protective nutritional supplements, and one's diet. It has been shown that alcohol use doubles the risk for developing liver cancer in people infected chronically with the hepatitis C virus. In the United States and Italy, alcohol abuse is the most common factor in liver cancer risk. Consuming 80 grams of alcohol a day for 10 years increases one's risk fivefold.

One of the big questions is—How long does one have to abstain from alcohol before their risk falls to that of a non-drinker? It has been estimated that one would have to abstain 23 years to reach that goal. One study found that risk falls 6 to 7% a year with abstaining. Taking nutrients and special liver protecting and repairing natural compounds, such as Nano-Silymarin, Nano-Curcumin, Nano-Quercetin, baicalin, and berberine, as well as B-complex vitamins, vitamin C, mixed tocopherols, taurine, and mixed tocotrienols, along with magnesium and zinc will go a long way in repairing the liver damage, reducing liver scarring (fibrosis), and preventing a liver cancer from developing.

Categories of Liver Cancer

There are two categories of liver tumors: benign tumors, which are generally harmless, and liver cancers, the dangerous type that spreads. The latter includes the hepatocellular carcinoma we have been discussing.

Benign Liver Tumors

Benign liver tumors are common. They do not spread to other areas of the body and they usually do not pose a serious health risk. In fact, most of the time, benign liver tumors do not cause any symptoms, so they are diagnosed "incidentally," which means they are found if you undergo a medical imaging test, such as an ultrasound, CT scan, or MRI, for another condition. Rarely do they require treatment.

The Three Kinds of Benign Liver Tumors

- **Hemangiomas.** Hemangiomas, which are masses of abnormal blood vessels, are the most common type of liver tumors. It's estimated that up to 5% of adults have small hemangiomas in their liver. They are more common in women. Usually, these benign tumors produce no symptoms and do not need to be treated. When symptoms do occur, either due to size or location, they may need to be surgically removed.
- **Focal nodular hyperplasias (FNHs).** These are the second most common form of benign liver tumors. These tumors do not cause symptoms or require treatment. They usually occur in women between the ages of 20 and 30. In very rare cases, if they are large or causing pain, they may need to be removed surgically.
- **Hepatocellular adenomas.** These are less common benign liver tumors, which occur most often in in women of childbearing age and have been linked to oral contraceptive use, where higher doses of estrogen were used. They rarely cause problems. They may also occur in women who take hormones. In these cases, women are advised to discontinue birth control pills or hormones to prevent further growth. In rare cases, surgery may be needed.

Metastatic Liver Cancer

Metastatic liver cancer is dangerous, because these tumors can invade and damage other tissues around them. They can also break off and spread (metastasize) to other parts of the body. Colorectal cancers, renal cell carcinoma, melanomas, pancreatic cancer, sarcomas, stomach cancer, lung cancers, and breast cancer are the types that most commonly spread to the liver.

Colorectal cancer is the most common type to spread to the liver. Approximately 50% of colorectal cancer patients will develop liver metastasis, and only a minority of these tumors can be successfully removed surgically. Recent studies indicate that around 40% will survive 5 years following removal of the liver tumor if the metastasis is a single tumor, as opposed to less than a 1% survival with multiple metastatic liver tumors.

Despite attempts at curative surgery to remove the tumor, approximately 65% will recur within the liver within 3 years, even with aggressive chemotherapy. Cryotherapy and radiofrequency ablation have slightly better results for all types of tumors and are less likely to spread tumor cells as opposed to open surgical resection of the tumor.

Types of Primary Liver Cancers

- **Hepatocellular carcinoma.** This type of liver cancer, known also as hepatoma, or HCC, is the most common type of liver cancer, accounting for three-quarters of all liver cancer. This type of cancer develops in the hepatocytes, which are the predominant liver cells. It can spread from the liver to other parts of the body, such as the pancreas, intestines, and stomach. It occurs much more often in people with severe liver damage of several types, especially with cirrhosis, but is particularly common with alcohol abuse. HCC-type tumors are most often diagnosed late in their course, with only 40% or less being diagnosed early. People who are diagnosed with an advanced form of this type of liver cancer have a very poor survival rate despite the best conventional treatment.

- **Cholangiocarcinoma.** More commonly known as bile duct cancer, this type of cancer is less common, accounting for up to 20% of all liver cancers. Cancer that begins inside the bile ducts within the liver is called *intrahepatic bile duct cancer*; when it begins in the section of the ducts outside the liver, it's called *extrahepatic bile duct cancer.*
- **Liver angiosarcoma.** This rare form of liver cancer begins in the blood vessels of the liver and tends to progress very quickly, so it is typically diagnosed at a more advanced stage.
- **Hepatoblastoma.** This extremely rare type of liver cancer is nearly always found in children, usually under age three.

Symptoms

Symptoms rarely occur in the early stages of liver cancer, so it may be advanced by the time it is discovered. When they do occur, symptoms can include:

- Abdominal discomfort, pain, and tenderness
- Jaundice
- White, chalky stools
- Nausea
- Vomiting
- Bruising or bleeding easily
- Weakness
- Fatigue

Is Liver Cancer Preventable?

Yes, many cases are preventable, as research published in 2018 in *CA: A Cancer Journal for Clinicians* suggests.

According to this one study, 71% of liver cancer diagnoses in the U.S. can be attributed to these preventable causes. Links to a high risk of liver cancer include:

- Hepatitis C, B, D, and HIV
- Excess body weight (obesity and overweight)
- Smoking
- Alcoholism
- Type 2 diabetes
- Metabolic syndrome
- Insulin resistance
- Nonalcoholic steatohepatitis–NASH (the severe form of fatty liver disease)
- Exposure to toxic liver compounds
  - Pesticides/herbicides
  - Industrial chemicals
  - Artificial sweeteners (aspartame, sucralose, and saccharine)
  - Excitotoxic food additives (MSG, hydrolyzed proteins, soy protein extracts, etc.)

"Basically, preventing exposure to those risk factors would mean a substantial proportion of liver cancer deaths—about 50%—could be prevented," says Farhad Islami, strategic director for cancer surveillance research at the American Cancer Society in Atlanta, who led the study. Using the more powerful natural liver protectants, such as Nano-Curcumin, Nano-Quercetin, baicalin, berberine, Nano-Silymarin, and apigenin would probably lower these risks even more.

Causes of Liver Cancer

- **Genetics.** Liver cancer is not technically an inherited disease; however, people who inherit the disease hereditary hemochromatosis may be prone to it. People with this disease absorb too much iron from their food. The iron accumulates in tissues throughout the body, predominantly in the liver. If enough iron builds up in the liver, it can lead to cirrhosis and liver cancer. Liver cancer is also more common with certain genetic markers, such as GTSM1 and PNPLA3. Wilson's disease is also associated with liver cirrhosis, with secondary to high levels of tissue copper.
- **Existing liver disease.** As noted, people with hereditary hemochromatosis are at increased risk. Also, hepatitis and Wilson's disease can progress to liver cancer. Hepatitis viruses can alter the liver's DNA by inducing chronic smoldering inflammation and making the liver more susceptible to cancer.
- **Alcohol use.** Alcohol abuse is a leading cause of cirrhosis in the U.S., which in turn is linked with an increased risk of liver cancer. Heavy drinkers have about double the risk of two types of liver cancer: hepatocellular carcinoma and intrahepatic cholangiocarcinoma.
- **Smoking.** Current smokers have a 51 to 70% increased liver cancer risk, and those who quit are still at increased risk, although less so. According to research, those who have quit smoking for 30 years or more are at no increased risk.
- **Type 2 diabetes.** This common form of diabetes is linked to an increased risk of liver cancer, usually because of other factors such as heavy alcohol use and/or chronic viral hepatitis. Also, people with type 2 diabetes tend to be overweight or obese, which in turn can cause liver problems.

- **Chemicals.** Exposure to certain chemicals can damage the liver. Chemicals in the workplace include vinyl chloride, which is used to make plastic, and thorium dioxide (Thorotrast), which is a chemical used in the past that was injected into patients as part of certain X-ray tests. Vinyl chloride is now tightly regulated and Thorotrast is no longer used. Arsenic, which can be found in drinking water, is also part of the process of making vinyl chloride, and is linked to liver damage and cancer risk. Aflaxtoxin, a chemical found in a type of fungus, is the reason for some liver cancer in Africa and other developing nations. As mentioned, even certain brand-name peanut butter contains some aflatoxins.
- **Anabolic steroids.** The long-term use of anabolic steroids, male hormones used by some athletes to increase their strength and muscle mass, can slightly increase hepatocellular cancer risk. Cortisone-like steroids, such as hydrocortisone, prednisone, and dexamethasone, do not carry this same risk.

Diagnosing Liver Cancer

If liver cancer is diagnosed at an early stage, the 5-year survival rate is 33%. If liver cancer has spread to surrounding tissues or organs and/or the regional lymph nodes, the 5-year survival rate is 11%. If the cancer has spread to a distant part of the body, the 5-year survival rate is only 2%. These figures include the use of conventional treatments. Based on several carefully done studies, combining conventional treatments with selected use of plant extracts can significantly improve survival and reduce the side effects of conventional treatments. Those not wishing to follow conventional treatment, which generally have had dismal results, may wish to use natural treatments only or a combination of the two as outlined in the following.

However, the problem with liver cancer is that too often cases go undiscovered until the cancer is at an advanced stage, mainly because symptoms appear early. One reason is because the liver, being a large organ, is late to demonstrate symptoms.

You should be screened for liver cancer if:

- You have a family history of liver cancer or cirrhosis.
- You have chronic hepatitis B or C.
- You have fatty liver disease.
- You have been exposed to known liver toxins.
- You drink more than three drinks a day every day.
- You are obese, especially if you have type 2 diabetes.
- You have hemochromatosis or Wilson's disease.

If you have other risk factors for liver disease, you should discuss test screenings with your doctor. Screening options include testing the blood for a substance called *alpha-fetoprotein* (AFP), which may be produced by cancer cells. AFP can also be elevated in 20 to 25% of patients having chronic cirrhosis, hepatitis, or other liver diseases. That is, it is not specific for liver cancer. Other diagnostic tests include imaging studies and non-invasive tests, such as an ultrasound, computed tomography (CT or CAT) scan, or magnetic resonance imaging (MRI). An MRI scan is the most accurate and uses no radiation.

Liver Cancer Treatment

Especially when diagnosed at an early stage, there are several potential treatments for hepatocellular carcinoma, the most common form of liver cancer.

There are two common surgeries used to treat this form of liver cancer:

Surgery

Surgery for liver cancer, known as partial hepatectomy, is likely to be the most successful disease-directed treatment, particularly if you have good liver function and tumors that can be safely removed from a limited portion of the liver. Surgery may not be an option if the tumor takes up too much of the liver, the liver is too damaged, the tumor has spread outside the liver, or the patient has other serious illnesses. With this surgery, the cancerous portion of the liver is removed, and the liver may regenerate or regrow the missing portion.

With early diagnosis, there is a 70% 5-year survival and 60% with a partial resection. Overall, the 5-year tumor recurrence rate is 20 to 35%.

Liver Transplant

In a liver transplant, the entire liver is removed and a liver from a donor will replace the diseased one. This procedure is possible only when specific criteria are met, including tumor size and number, and whether a suitable donor is found. Liver transplantation is a particularly effective treatment for people with a small tumor because transplantation removes the tumor and the damaged liver. However, there are few donors, and you may have to wait a long time before a liver becomes available. With liver transplantation, there is a 15% chance of tumor recurrence in the new organ.

Nonsurgical Treatments

Radiotherapy Ablation

Known also as thermal ablation, this minimally invasive treatment uses a tiny needle to destroy the tumor with microwave directed heat. This treatment can be administered through the skin, through laparoscopy, or during a surgical operation.

Cryotherapy

This also uses a small probe percutaneously (through the skin) to freeze the tumor, which not only kills the tumor but also prevents seeding of the tumor cells, which occurs extensively with open surgery. Studies have shown that freezing the tumor also stimulates an immune attack on any residual tumor cells. Results in most treatment series are superior to other forms of treatment.

Stereotactic Body Radiation Therapy (SBRT)

This treatment applies high doses of radiation therapy to a tumor while limiting the amount of radiation to nearby healthy tissue. Performed to treat tumors that are about 5 cm or smaller.

Advanced Liver Cancer Treatments

The following treatments are considered in advanced liver cancer:

Chemotherapy

Chemotherapy is the utilization of certain drugs to destroy cancer cells, usually by keeping the cancer cells from growing, dividing, and making more cells. For this procedure, called *chemo-embolization*, drugs are injected into the hepatic artery (the vessel that supplies blood to the liver), blocking the flow for a short time so the chemotherapy stays in the tumor longer. These treatments have been very disappointing and associated with serious complications.

Radioembolization

This procedure is similar to chemoembolization, except that it involves the placement of radioactive beads into the artery that supplies the tumor with blood. The beads deliver radiation therapy directly into the tumor when they become trapped in the small blood vessels of the tumor. Results have been less than stellar.

Targeted Treatments

Targeted therapies are drugs that target the cancer's specific genes, proteins, or the tissue environment that contributes to cancer growth and survival. This type of treatment blocks the growth and spread of cancer cells while limiting damage to healthy cells. So far they have added little to the overall treatment.

Immunotherapy

Also called *biologic therapy*, immunotherapy uses the body's immune system to help fight the cancer. One common type of immunotherapy is called an *immune checkpoint inhibitor*. Immune checkpoint inhibitors work by blocking the pathways that would otherwise allow the cancer to hide from the immune system. These treatments probably have a greater chance of success, but also can have significant side effects that can be prolonged.

Natural Treatments That Have Shown Significant Experimental Results

Why Natural Anticancer Compounds Are Better

Unknown to most physicians, there exists extensive, carefully conducted, scientific studies on a growing number of natural compounds, most extracted from plants, demonstrating powerful and far safer ways to combat many cancers, including liver cancer.

By attacking several mechanisms essential for cancer growth and invasion of surrounding tissues, natural compounds like berberine, curcumin, quercetin, and baicalin, demonstrate far better anticancer effectiveness than most chemotherapy drugs. Most chemotherapy drugs attack only one aspect of the cancer cell, which most cancer cells can quickly overcome. We call this multidrug resistance (MDR), a process that accounts for most failures of drug treatments for cancer. When MDR occurs, the cancer becomes resistant to all other chemotherapy drugs.

Interestingly, natural anticancer compounds only damage cancer cells and do not damage normal cells, something chemotherapy drugs cannot do—they damage all cells, cancerous and normal. This explains why chemotherapy drugs cause so many side effects. In fact, natural anticancer compounds help protect the surrounding normal cells and tissues from damage by chemotherapy and radiation therapy.

Most patients are told to avoid these natural compounds because the cancer doctor fears these natural compounds may interfere with their chemotherapy treatments. Extensive studies have not only shown this not to be true, but in many cases the natural compounds actually make the chemotherapy drugs much more effective in killing cancer cells than when the drug is used alone. That is, the natural compounds enhance the effectiveness of the conventional treatments.

In addition, extensive studies have shown that most of these natural compounds are extremely safe, even in very large doses. And, as mentioned, these natural products can dramatically reduce the side effects of chemotherapy and radiotherapy.

Because most practicing physicians, even those who specialize in cancer (oncologists), never read these research articles, so they are unaware of these facts, they don't know that these compounds are backed by extensive scientific studies by some of the best experts and laboratories in the world. Unfortunately, most medical universities are controlled by big pharmaceutical company money, which discourages teaching about these natural treatments.

Berberine

Berberine is an extract from the roots of several plants, such as barberry and goldenseal. Extensive studies have demonstrated numerous mechanisms by which this extract kills and inhibits liver cancer growth and invasion. One principal way berberine inhibits cancer development and growth of existing tumors is by inhibiting liver inflammation. It does this by inhibiting the receptors used by the immune system to cause liver inflammation (mainly TLR4). Berberine has also been shown to powerfully inhibit the release of interferon and several inflammatory cytokines (TNF, IL-6, and IL1ß).

Studies on tumor cells and human tumors transplanted into animals have shown berberine to be effective in inhibiting several types of cancer, such as breast, lung, colon, and liver cancers. A recent study found a very powerful mechanism by which berberine suppresses and kills cancer cells.

It has been known for a very long time that cancer cells metabolize energy sources differently than normal cells. Newer treatments of cancer have utilized this knowledge with great success in many cancers, even highly malignant tumors. Extensive studies have shown that cancer cells consume glutamine in very high concentrations and are, in fact, dependent on high concentrations of glutamine to survive.

Once inside the cancer cell, the glutamine is converted into glutamate, the excitotoxic amino acid. Glutamate has been shown to make most cancer cells grow much faster and become more invasive. One can think of glutamine and glutamate as cancer fertilizers.

A recent study found that berberine blocks the transporter that allows glutamine to enter the cancer cell, essentially starving these dangerous cells. This lowers both glutamine and glutamate levels in liver cancer cells. In part of the study, researchers used actual human liver cancers grown in mice. They then fed the mice berberine and found a dramatic reduction in the size of the tumors.

That glutamine is essential for liver cancer growth was further demonstrated when researchers found that liver cancers with high levels of the glutamine transporter had the poorest prognosis, and those with the lowest levels had prolonged survivals. The researchers also found that the cancer gene called *c-myc* controlled the glutamine transporter. Patients with high levels of c-myc in their tumors had the worse prognosis. Interestingly, berberine suppresses this cancer gene, thereby reducing glutamine access to the tumor.

The main problem with berberine is that it is poorly absorbed from the GI tract. The Nano-Berberine form is far better absorbed and would be expected to be more effective in inhibiting liver cancer. Nano-Berberine can be purchased at One Planet Nutrition Company. I have no financial connection to this company, but I use their products. The usual dose would be 500 mg taken three times a day with or without meals.

Baicalin

Another plant extract of great interest in inhibiting liver damage and liver cancer is baicalin, an extract from the plant *Scutellaria baicalensis Georgi*, also known as skullcap. You might see articles making reference to baicalein, which is a chemical relative of baicalin. In fact, once consumed, baicalein is converted in the body to baicalin, the active ingredient.

Baicalin has powerful antiviral effects against hepatitis viruses, mainly by preventing the virus from replicating. Combining baicalin with a component found in tea, called *catechin*, powerfully inhibits hepatitis B virus replication, rendering it harmless. Combining baicalin with other antiviral drugs has been shown to also suppress hepatitis B virus from replicating and potently reduces liver inflammation, which significantly lowers one's risk of developing liver cancer.

Other ways baicalin reduces the risk of liver cancer is by suppressing fat accumulation in the liver, and most importantly, by reducing fibrosis of the liver, the beginning stage of liver cirrhosis. This extract also reduces obesity, lowers serum triglycerides, reduces total cholesterol, lowers small dense LDL levels, and reduces elevated liver enzymes (indicating the repair of liver damage). If this is not enough, baicalin also increases the level of liver glutathione and SOD enzyme, two powerful antioxidants. It also inhibits inflammation directly and reduces insulin resistance, thereby reducing the risk of developing type 2 diabetes.

Studies have also shown that baicalin reduces iron overload in the liver (and other organs and tissues), reduces liver damage by acetaminophen, and reduces toxicity by various liver-damaging chemicals. Baicalin has also been shown to significantly reduce liver damage due to alcohol abuse and enhances liver function.

For people already having liver cancer, baicalin has been shown to inhibit the growth of the tumor, increase the killing of tumor cells by the immune system, and stimulate autophagy, a process used by the cells to kill cancer cells.

In general, baicalin has a high safety margin and is well-tolerated, even in doses as high as 2800 mg a day. It is also used to enhance memory and learning.

Unfortunately, baicalin is poorly absorbed. There is a finely powdered form that comes in either a loose powder or capsule form. One can mix the loose powder in 4 ounces of water and drink it. I prefer to do this because I think it improves absorption. It should be taken at least 30 minutes before a meal and taken with 1000 mg of vitamin C to prevent excess iron chelation (removal). If you have a high iron level and want to remove iron, take it with meals and avoid taking the vitamin C at the same time. The usual dose is 250 mg three times a day.

Quercetin (Nano-Quercetin)

Quercetin is a flavonoid commonly found in teas, onions, and many vegetables. Studies have shown quercetin to have very powerful liver protective properties and to enhance liver repair and function when used in moderate doses. In fact, one of the animal models they used induced severe liver damage using carbon tetrachloride (previously used in fire extinguishers). The quercetin dramatically protected the liver from damage and helped restore normal liver function. One way quercetin protects the liver is to reduce high levels of nitric oxide, which when elevated causes intense inflammation and tissue destruction.

It is also known that people with cirrhosis can develop severe lung damage as well. One study found that quercetin could dramatically protect against this damage. Again, quercetin protected the lungs by reducing elevated nitric oxide levels in the arteries supplying the lungs.

Several studies have shown that quercetin reduces fat accumulation in the liver, thus protecting against both NAFLD and the more serious type, NASH. There is evidence that one way quercetin helps the liver is by protecting the probiotic balance of organisms in the colon. This has been shown to reduce liver fat accumulation and inflammation in the liver.

Quercetin has also been shown to protect against insulin sensitivity and glucose intolerance even when animals are fed a fatty diet. This flavonoid also improved gut barrier function (preventing leaky gut), increased the production of short-chain fatty acids (SCFAs), and reduced the level of several inflammatory cytokines. Butyrate, one of the SCFAs, is important in preventing colon cancer and in repairing a leaky gut.

NASH, nonalcoholic steatohepatitis, is a much more serious condition than just a simple fatty liver (NAFLD), in that there exists widespread inflammation in the liver, which increases the risk of liver fibrosis, cirrhosis, and liver cancer. Quercetin has been shown to be a major weapon against NASH and instrumental in preventing liver cancer in people with NASH.

Another, less common cause for liver cirrhosis is obstruction of the bile ducts used in draining the bile from the liver. When the bile backs up in the liver, it can trigger intense inflammation and scarring. One study found that quercetin could dramatically reduce the damage to the liver caused by this obstruction, including the scarring (fibrosis).

Obstruction of the bile ducts causes a severe loss of vitamin E, glutathione, and high levels of nitric oxide within the liver. Quercetin lowered the excess nitric oxide and raised glutathione levels. Vitamin E should be replaced using mixed tocopherols in a dose of 400 IU twice a day with meals. Mixed tocotrienols should also be taken in a dose of 100 mg a day with a meal.

Because quercetin is so poorly absorbed, a Nano-Quercetin product has been developed, which is far better absorbed and distributed in the body tissues. Moderate doses should be used because extremely high doses have been shown to cause some DNA damage.

The dose of Nano-Quercetin is 250 mg taken three times a day with a meal. It can cause reactive hypoglycemia, so it should always be taken with food.

Silymarin (Nano-Silymarin)

Silymarin, a group of compounds found in the milk thistle plant, has been used to protect and treat a number of liver conditions. Extensive animal and human studies have confirmed the effectiveness and safety of this group of flavonoids.

This compound has been shown to be very effective in protecting the liver from alcohol damage and in repairing much of this damage. Excessive alcohol intake rapidly depletes the liver's antioxidant vitamins, B-complex vitamins, and triggers intense inflammation throughout the liver.

One of the more impressive studies, mentioned previously, used 12 baboons that were fed a diet composed of 50% alcohol for 36 months. The researchers performed a liver biopsy every 6 months throughout the study to evaluate the liver damage. They also measured levels of liver enzymes, total bilirubin, triglycerides, and collagen (to evaluate fibrosis). The alcohol progressively damaged the animals' livers, which appeared as abnormal in liver tests and histology. The animals given the silymarin demonstrated a dramatic reduction in powerful free radicals, the liver enzyme ALT returned to normal, and most importantly there was a dramatic reduction in liver fibrosis. All of the animals given the silymarin were significantly protected and two out of six of the baboons were fully protected when examined 3 years after the study ended.

The usual dose of Nano-Silymarin for prevention of damage would be 250 mg three times a day with meals. Higher doses would be used to treat established liver disorders, such as 500 mg three times a day with meals.

Apigenin

Apigenin is a flavonoid found in abundance in several plants, including celery, parsley, artichokes, and chamomile. Supplements are available containing concentrations of this flavonoid. Studies have shown a very high level of safety with apigenin use. Nanosized apigenin is not commercially available yet. Absorption is increased by taking the supplement with food.

As we have seen throughout this book, fibrosis and associated inflammation are the two main triggers for developing liver cancer. Things that inhibit these two conditions drastically reduce the risk. A recent study found that the cells producing the fibrosis (scarring) are hepatic stellate cells, which release a compound strongly linked to liver fibrosis called TGF-ß1. In this study, the researchers used a low-dose and a high-dose of apigenin in animal models of severe liver disease.

They found that the apigenin significantly reduced the amount of fibrosis in the animals' livers, mainly by dramatically reducing the level of TGF-ß1 being released from the stellate cells of the liver. Further, they demonstrated that the beneficial effects were dose-related, meaning the higher the dose of apigenin, the better the protection.

Another study found that apigenin lowered the level of fats in the blood, reduced liver inflammation and inflammatory cytokines, decreased insulin resistance, and reduced total cholesterol and markers for atherosclerosis risks.

Studies have also shown that curcumin can significantly reduce liver fibrosis and inflammation by lowering TGF-ß1.

Combining Nano-Curcumin and apigenin will dramatically increase this protection. One study demonstrated that highly absorbable apigenin significantly inhibited the development of liver cancer in animal models with severe liver damage and fibrosis. Apigenin has been shown to restore the level of all the antioxidant enzymes, vitamin C, and vitamin E, as well as gluta-thione—all things that significantly reduce the risk of developing a liver cancer and that restore liver health.

Green Tea Extract

While components of green and white teas can suppress primary liver cancer (hepatocellular carcinoma), one study found that when combined with a low dose of the chemotherapy agent doxorubicin, there was a profound inhibition of this form of cancer. Doxorubicin is the most commonly used drug to treat this cancer, but because it has such a toxic effect on the body, especially the liver and heart, it cannot be used in doses high enough to offer a significant benefit. This study found that by combining it with extracts of green and white teas called ECG (epicatechin gallate) and EGCG (epigallocatechin gallate), very small doses of the chemotherapy drug (doxorubicin) could be used (that had few side effects, but powerful anticancer effectiveness). Other studies have shown this to be true of all chemotherapy—one can use much smaller doses if combined with anticancer plant flavonoids with even greater effectiveness, fewer side effects, and safety.

In this study, they were testing a form of resistant hepato-cellular carcinoma that was highly resistant to all chemotherapy drugs (called *multidrug resistance*). The tea extract made the cancer highly sensitive to the drug. The benefit of the tea extract was that it stimulated higher levels of the drug entering the cancer cells. With MDR, a special compound (P-gp) keeps the chemotherapy drug out of the cancer cell, which prevents the drug from killing the cancer cells.

The problem with most cases of hepatocellular carcinoma is that the tumor develops MDR very rapidly. Using conventional treatments, most patients die in less than a year. By adding the tea catechins and lower doses of chemotherapy drugs, one can expect a much higher survival rate and possibly a higher cure rate. White and green tea extracts also significantly reduce strokes.

There have been rare cases of severe liver failure in people taking just small doses of the extracts or even drinking green tea. These cases are extremely rare and once the tea is stopped, the liver usually recovers.

Combatting Liver Metastasis Using Natural Compounds

One of the most impressive anticancer treatments I have researched utilizes a combination of myoinositol and inositol-6 phosphate (IP6). Earlier studies have shown that this combination was quite powerful in inhibiting the development of chemically induced liver cancers in animal models—a standard way to study liver cancers. It appears that severely damaged livers, associated with a high risk of liver cancer, have a common severe defect in a cellular compound called *glutathione-S-transferase*. The combination of myoinositol and IP6 markedly increases the concentration of this essential compound in liver cells, thus suppressing the development of liver cancer. Both compounds are potent inhibitors of hepatocellular carcinomas.

One of the most common metastatic cancers traveling to the liver is colorectal cancer, which can appear as a single metastatic tumor or many such tumors scattered throughout the liver. Using a special animal model of metastatic colorectal cancer that imitates what we see in people with colorectal cancer spread, researchers found that the animals receiving the combination of myoinositol and IP6 had the greatest shrinkage of the liver metastasis, with less shrinkage when the two compounds were used alone.

Intense study revealed that the supplement compounds in combination suppressed a cancer cell signaling process essential for cancer growth and progression. IP6, in other studies, has been shown to effectively kill several types of cancer cells, such as prostate cancer, melanoma, and breast and colon cancers. Other studies have shown that myoinositol plus IP6 inhibit many essential cancer cell mechanisms.

In one animal study of colorectal cancer metastasis, researchers demonstrated that, in untreated mice, the liver metastatic tumors occupied the entire liver. Those treated with the myoinositol alone or the IP6 alone had some shrinkage of the liver cancer, but the combination dramatically shrunk the tumor, and extensively reduced the number of cancer blood vessels in the tumors (called *angiogenesis*, a process essential to cancer growth and survival). The combination of the two products caused a 72.5% shrinkage of the liver tumor.

In another study, in which human liver cancer cells (HepG2 cells) were implanted in mice, scientists found that the mice given IP6 developed no tumors, whereas 71% of the animals given no IP6 developed cancerous tumors in the liver.

Another powerful inhibitor of metastatic liver cancer is green tea compounds (even higher levels of these anticancer compounds are in white tea). A Japanese study found that taking a supplement containing a green tea powder concentrate equal to 10 cups of green tea, reduced the recurrence of colorectal adenocarcinoma by 52%. Combining the green tea compound EGCG with conventional treatment reduced tumor volume by 70.3%, a very dramatic result.

Another tumor that commonly metastasizes to the liver is the melanoma-type cancers. One very interesting study found that a combination of myoinositol and IP6 completely cured a grade IV melanoma in a patient who could not take conventional treatments. The patient had widespread metastatic tumors before he started the combination of anticancer compounds. He was completely tumor-free 3 years after the article was published.

One of the most important breakthroughs in cancer research is the discovery that all cancers seem to arise from **cancer stem cells,** and that the bulk of the cancer is composed of cells (daughter cells) that are far less cancerous and dangerous. Most traditional treatments only kill the daughter cells and not the main culprit, the cancer stem cells, which can make up only 1 to 10% of the volume of the tumor.

The cancer stem cell can be thought of as a child's bubble blower, which blows thousands of bubbles and even more if you blow harder. The bubbles represent the main bulk of the tumor composed of the daughter cells. You can remove all the bubbles (resembling chemotherapy and radiotherapy), but in a very short period they will all reappear—resembling the reoccurrence of the cancer. Unfortunately, cancer stem cells are resistant to most conventional drugs and treatments, which explains the dismal long-term cure rate seen in many cancer patients.

Ironically, several natural anticancer compounds powerfully inhibit and kill cancer stem cells, such as curcumin, quercetin, and pterostilbene. In fact, a recent study demonstrated the ability of pterostilbene and blueberry extracts (high in pterostilbene) to kill cancer stem cells. The study also found that the extracts made the cancers much more sensitive to radiation treatments.

Final Words

When I was still practicing neurosurgery, I was dabbling in nutrition studies and doing my best to pull together as many studies on nutrition as possible—which in the days before the internet was no easy task, and was very time consuming.

While making rounds in the hospital, a nurse approached me, knowing I had an interest in nutrition, and told me her husband was suffering from hepatitis C, was bedridden, and had been so for several months. He was quite depressed about his fate, having been told he may not be able to work anytime soon. The couple were in their early to mid-twenties. I wrote out some suggestions based on my research and later forgot about the whole episode.

One day, my wife and I were out shopping when the same nurse approached me with her husband. After introductions were exchanged, he thanked me for what I had done for him and stated that he was back to his old self, full of energy and feeling great. The program I outlined for him quickly restored his health and he now had his life back. His wife expressed her gratitude as well and reminded me that his doctors had little hope for his improvement.

Unfortunately, traditional medicine has advanced very little since then—which was over 25 years ago. If a prescription drug is not available, the doctor is at a loss as to what can be done. Most doctors are unaware of the extensive research being done on natural compounds. From my studies, most liver disorders can be dramatically improved, and most of the dreadful complications avoided, chiefly through the use of simple natural methods and natural compounds. In most instances, these compounds have a wide margin of safety.

CHAPTER 17

Liver Transplantation

Over the past 40 years or so, liver transplants have become an accepted way of treating certain chronic and acute conditions that cause severe and irreversible liver dysfunction. Next to the kidney, the liver is the most commonly transplanted organ, followed by the heart and lung, in that order.

A liver transplant is performed by using a whole liver or a partial liver taken from a donor, either living or deceased, which is used to replace the recipient's diseased liver. The surgical procedure is complex and depends on the careful harvesting of the organ from the donor, as well as successful implementation in the recipient.

Such a procedure is major surgery, which carries risks, and requires the recipient to take antirejection drugs.

In 2017, about 8000 liver transplants were performed in the U.S. among both adults and children. Of those, about 360 involved livers from living donors. At the same time, approximately 11,500 people were registered on the waiting list for a liver transplant.

Who Are Liver Transplant Candidates?

If you have liver disease that has advanced beyond regular treatment, you'll be referred to a specialized liver transplant center for further evaluation. This evaluation usually takes place over the course of a few days, and is done to determine whether you are eligible for a liver transplant. Once the evaluation is complete, you'll be placed on a waiting list.

Not all people with liver problems are deemed suitable candidates for surgery. The recipient needs to be carefully chosen, to help increase the odds for a successful surgery.

Liver transplants have a high success rate in treating cirrhosis, chronic hepatitis, liver cancer, and other forms of advanced or irreversible liver disease. However, people with diseases originating outside the liver, or those that have spread beyond the liver are generally not deemed good candidates. An ongoing alcohol or drug problem can also rule out a transplant, as can poor health, especially serious heart or lung problems.

However, although patients with some types of liver diseases are not deemed appropriate immediately, they could become candidates should their conditions change.

How Successful Are Liver Transplants?

Your chances of a successful liver transplant and long-term survival depend on a great many factors. It also depends on the skill and experience of the surgical team. Success rates vary widely and are dependent on many complex factors, not all of it under the control of the transplant team. For example, the incidence of acute rejection of the transplanted liver varies from 24 to 80%, depending on these complex factors.

Mortality within the first year after the transplant usually occurs within the first 3 months, and is most often due to infection, primary graft failure, rejection of the organ, and technical complications. Later mortality is usually due to such factors as cardiovascular disease, malignancy, infections, chronic organ rejection and graft failure, and chronic kidney failure. The most common cause of death following a liver transplant is attributed to problems associated with immunosuppression or complications associated with the drugs used to suppress rejection immunity.

Success also depends on the reason for the transplant, such as cryptogenic cirrhosis, viral hepatitis, alcoholic cirrhosis, or exposure to toxic chemicals. Approximately 95% of people undergoing liver transplants for viral hepatitis will have the virus present in the new liver and their blood. Despite this high incidence of viral infection, less than half will show clinical signs of the infection, and about 20 to 40% will progress to cirrhosis of the new liver within 5 years. One of the major problems is that having to use immunosuppressive drugs in the face of a viral infection greatly increases the persistence of the virus. For example, one study found that using corticosteroids to prevent organ rejection problems resulted in a 4-fold to 100-fold increase in positive test results for the presence of the virus in the blood.

Patients with end-stage liver disease secondary to alcoholic cirrhosis in some studies were in poorer health, younger, and required re-operation more often than for other causes. One of the major risks with alcoholic cirrhosis is a resumption of alcohol use after the transplant, which will damage the new liver. With the use of natural products known to protect the liver in such cases, the incidence of these problems would be much less.

It has also been found that patients who received the immune stimulant drug alpha-interferon had a much higher rate of rejection of the new liver than those not needing the drug. This drug is a standard treatment used in treating viral hepatitis.

In general, about 75% of people who undergo liver transplant live for at least 5 years. That means that for every 100 people who receive a liver transplant for any reason, about 75 will live for 5 years and 30 will die within 5 years.

People who receive a liver from a living donor often have better short-term survival rates than those who receive a deceased-donor liver, but that could be because these recipients aren't as sick as those who receive a deceased-donor liver because their wait for an organ is shorter.

These are the most recent survival rates for people with liver transplants from deceased donors, according to the NIH's National Institute of Diabetes and Digestive and Kidney Diseases:

- 86% at 1 year
- 78% at 3 years
- 72% at 5 years
- 53% at 20 years

More information on survival rates among liver transplant recipients also varies among U.S. transplant centers and can be found online at the Scientific Registry of Transplant Recipients.

Three Types of Liver Transplant

Deceased-Donor Transplants

Most livers for transplants come from people who have just died, which are called *cadaveric donations*. In a cadaveric donation transplantation, surgeons remove the diseased or injured liver and replace it with the deceased donor's liver. Adults typically receive the entire liver from a deceased donor. However, surgeons may split a deceased donor's liver into two parts. The larger part may go to an adult, and the smaller part may go to a smaller adult or child.

When a donated liver becomes available, the first patients to be considered are those who are determined to be most in need within the shortest distance of the donor. The donor liver is tested for viruses and also for compatibility. The liver transplant must be done quickly, because the organ can remain viable for only a limited number of hours.

Living-Donor Liver Transplants

Sometimes, a healthy living person will donate part of his or her liver, most often to a family member who is recommended for a liver transplant. A liver from a living donor is a more recent procedure, and one that is less commonly done, but, when possible, it offers many advantages. The first is that the donor is usually someone who is personally known or related to the recipient. The wait is much shorter compared to that for a deceased donor, meaning that the recipient is likely to be in better health, reducing the risk of complications, and there is a better probability of the transplant being successful.

During a living-donor transplant, surgeons remove a part of the living donor's healthy liver and use it to replace the patient's diseased or injured liver. The living donor's liver grows back to normal size soon after the surgery. The part of the liver received also grows to normal size. Living-donor transplants are less common than deceased-donor transplants.

Although the number of transplants done from livingdonors is a small portion of the total, this number is growing.

Domino Liver Transplants

Another, less common, type of living-donor liver transplant is called a *domino liver transplant*. In a domino liver transplant, you receive a liver from a living donor who has a disease called *familial amyloidosis*. Familial amyloidosis is a very rare disorder in which an abnormal protein accumulates and eventually damages the body's internal organs.

The donor with familial amyloidosis receives a liver transplant to treat his or her condition. Then, the donor can give his or her liver to you in a domino liver transplant because the liver still functions well. You may eventually develop symptoms of amyloidosis, but these symptoms usually take decades to develop.

Recipients for this type of transplant are usually 55 years old or older and aren't expected to develop symptoms before the end of their natural life expectancy.

Who Is Eligible for a Liver Transplant?

Generally, there are two situations in which patients who have advanced liver disease find themselves. There are emergency cases, which need to be evaluated for transplant immediately, and there are chronic cases in which liver function deteriorates gradually. These are the people who more commonly need liver transplants.

Most commonly, people referred for liver transplants are those with a worsening chronic disease who have been under a doctor's care for a long time. Many of the conditions discussed earlier in this book fall into this category, including:

- Fatty liver disease (nonalcoholic steatohepatitis)
- Chronic viral hepatitis B and C
- Alcoholic liver disease
- Some types of liver cancer

- Certain autoimmune and genetic diseases
- Vascular diseases of the liver

People with acute, or sudden liver disease, may also require a transplant. This usually occurs if the person has ingested a toxin, or poison, or experienced an overdose. Acute hepatitis, or a blockage of the liver's blood vessels can also result in the need for a sudden liver transplant.

Those people who are usually not deemed to be candidates for a liver transplant are those whose current drinking or drug use could damage the new liver. Often, a six-month period of alcohol abstinence is required. Likewise, those with a current history of active drug abuse would not be considered.

In addition, someone with organ disease, such as advanced heart disease, might not be considered eligible because the person needs to be able to tolerate the stress involved in a transplant procedure.

Gender Differences in Liver Transplantation

There is a gender gap in liver transplantation. Men generally get transplants more often, spend a shorter time on waiting lists, and have more successful outcomes, according to a review in the *Journal of Hepatology*. This difference is most pronounced in transplants done because of hepatitis C, the study notes.

This research, in which several studies were reviewed, found that the most transplants in recipients in either gender were between 50 and 64 years of age.

The study found that women were 30% less likely than men to receive a transplant within 3 years of being placed on a waiting list. In addition, women were 9% less likely to receive transplants from living donors, and they were more likely to become at higher risk of death or too sick to receive one as well.

Research is ongoing to try to find reasons for the disparity between genders in liver transplants.

The Liver Transplant Center

Once it is determined that you are no longer treatable by medical means, you will be referred to a specialized liver transplant center for further evaluation.

The Liver Transplant Program is a multidisciplinary practice within the Transplant Center. There, you'll find a team consisting of doctors who specialize in liver diseases (hepatologists), transplantation surgeons, desk clinical assistants, transplant nurse coordinators, physician assistants, social workers, and dietitians, as well as other specialists that are utilized before, after, and during the transplant.

There are over 100 liver transplant centers in the U.S., including some that are attached to university medical schools.

Once you select a liver transplant center, you will go there for an evaluation. There, you will meet members of your center's transplant team, and you will also be evaluated according to such aspects as your physical, mental, financial, and social condition.

In addition, you'll be asked questions about your social support network, because a liver transplant requires a considerable recuperation period.

For the evaluation, you will undergo extensive medical testing to determine the extent of your liver disease, how well your liver functions, and the overall functioning of your body.

Whenever possible, the team will also evaluate whether there are any other ways to treat your liver disease, to avoid doing a liver transplant too early. Also, if alcohol is involved in your liver disease, you may need a referral to counseling or a rehabilitation program.

When considering a liver transplant center, the following is the information you need to know:

- Whether the center is located close to where you live.
- How many liver transplants are performed each year, and what the patient survival rates are. Experience counts, so large volume centers usually have better success rates. This is not always true as the surgeons' skill is more important than numbers of transplants done. A surgeon who does a large number of transplants poorly is of less value than one who does fewer well.
- What the cost is, whether your health insurance covers it, and what, if any, copayment is required. This includes costs incurred before, during, and after the transplant, as well as the travel arrangements, and the costs associated with housing during your recovery if you need to stay near the center, etc.
- Whether the center keeps up to date on the latest transplant research, technology, and techniques.

More Information

You can learn what liver transplant centers are located closest to you, and compare the number of procedures and success rates through the Scientific Registry of Transplant Recipients (www.srtr.org).

Liver Transplant Benefits and Risks

A liver transplant is a complicated procedure that affords great benefits, including improved survival and quality of life, but it also carries risks, including surgical complications, the possibility of recurrent liver disease, and a lifelong need to take immunosuppression drugs to prevent the liver from being rejected. The liver, though, is such an important organ to your well-being that, by the time liver disease is advanced, the benefits of a liver transplant usually outweigh the risk.

Risks of Liver Transplantation

- Bile duct complications, including bile duct leaks or shrinking of the bile ducts
- Bleeding
- Blood clots
- Failure of the donated liver
- Infection
- Rejection of the donated liver
- Mental confusion or seizures

Risks of Anti-rejection Drugs

- Bone thinning
- Diabetes
- Diarrhea
- Headaches
- High blood pressure
- High cholesterol

Waiting for a Liver Transplant

The wait for a liver from a deceased donor varies, but as of 2017, it was 239 days, according to the National Foundation for Transplants, which is an advocacy organization.

If you are a candidate for a liver transplant, your name will be added to a national database developed by the United Network for Organ Sharing (UNOS). Their website also provides excellent information about the transplantation process (www.unos.org).

Because of the lack of donor livers, in the past, controversies have emerged over livers given to famous or well-known recipients, including Mickey Mantle and Steve Jobs, to name two.

In 2019, the Organ Procurement and Transplantation Network (OPTN) was implemented to improve the process of matching liver and intestinal organs to candidates with the greatest need for them.

This goal of the new system is to save lives by providing more transplant access for the most urgent candidates. The new system replaced the use of decades-old geographic boundaries of 58 donation service areas (DSAs) and 11 transplant regions.

The final decision is based on a system called the Model for End-Stage Liver Disease (MELD), which was developed by UNOS to determine the severity of the disease for patients waiting on a liver transplant. The MELD score ranges from 6 to 40, with the most gravely ill patients having the highest numbers.

The MELD score assesses how sick the liver is, and the sicker the liver is, the higher the number, which means you are closer to a transplant. Race, sex, or ethnic background play no role in determining allocation of the organs. A person's spot on the waiting list depends on the availability of organs, the patient's blood type, and the medical urgency as reflected by their MELD score.

There are extra points for emergency requirements such as hepatocellular carcinoma, which is the most common type of liver cancer.

The MELD score usually increases as the liver disease worsens in the person on the waiting list. A MELD score can predict the 3-month and 1-year mortality, or the risk of death in most patients with chronic liver disease.

In very urgent cases, such as with drug overdose and acute liver failure, decisions for transplantation have to be made in a matter of days such as being over age 65 years with other serious illnesses, severe organ damage from other chronic diseases (such as diabetes), continuing to use alcohol or hepatotoxic drugs, or having irreversible brain damage.

There is a procedure similar to MELD that is used for pediatric patients.

The Liver Transplant Procedure

This is a brief explanation of what is involved in a liver transplant.

In the event you are receiving a liver from a deceased donor, you'll be asked to come to the hospital immediately. Your health care team will admit you to the hospital, and you'll undergo an exam to make sure you're healthy enough for the surgery.

Liver transplant surgery is done using general anesthesia, so you'll be sedated during the procedure. The transplant surgeon will make a long incision across your abdomen to access your liver.

Your surgeon will remove the diseased liver and place the donor liver in your body. Then the surgeon connects your blood vessels and bile ducts to the donor liver. Once your new liver is in place, the surgeon uses stitches and staples to close the surgical incision. You're then taken to the intensive care unit to begin recovery.

If you're receiving a liver transplant from a living donor, your surgery will be scheduled in advance. The surgeon will first operate on the donor, removing the portion of the liver for transplant. Then surgeons remove your diseased liver and place the donated liver portion in your body. They then connect your blood vessels and bile ducts to the new liver.

The transplanted liver portion in your body and the portion left behind in the donor's body regenerate rapidly, reaching normal volume within several weeks. Regardless of what type of transplant you have, it generally takes about 3 to 6 months to recuperate from a liver transplant.

After a Liver Transplant

After a liver transplant, you'll have to do everything you can to keep your new liver healthy. Here are recommendations from the National Institute of Diabetes and Digestive and Kidney Diseases:

- Take medicines exactly as your doctor tells you to take them.
- Talk with your doctor before taking any other medicines, including prescription and over-the-counter medicines, vitamins, and dietary supplements.
- Keep all medical appointments and scheduled blood draws.
- Stay away from people who are sick.
- Tell your doctor when you are sick.
- Learn to recognize the symptoms of rejection.
- Have cancer screenings as recommended by your doctor.
- Talk to your doctor, both before and after your liver transplant, about the use of contraceptives and the risks and outcomes of pregnancy.

A Special Note Concerning Diet and Liver Transplantation

The two major reasons for failure of a liver transplant include infection and immune rejection of the liver. First, one important animal study using rats in which 90% of the liver was removed, found that the mortality in rats fed a routine diet was 100% within 30 hours of the operation, whereas the rats fed a diet containing high levels of omega-3 oils had a 100% survival at 30 hours. Two weeks after the surgery, 20% of the rats given the omega-3 oil were still alive and all the rats on the regular diet had died.

Incredibly, the rats receiving the omega-3 oil demonstrated significant regeneration of their livers, along with restoration of the special architecture of the liver. Further study demonstrated that the special-fed rats had much higher levels of two cytokines that reduce liver inflammation and immune rejection: IL-4 and IL-10. This would also help prevent liver rejection.

Of more importance is a study that used patients who had liver transplants. In one such study, researchers studied 66 patients with end-stage liver disease or liver cancer undergoing a liver transplant. The patients were randomly divided into two groups of 33. Both groups were given a usual hospital diet for 7 days after their transplant surgery. One group, after the 7-day period, was given a special omega-3 oil emulsion. They were followed for 28 days for the study. The group getting the omega-3 oils had a dramatic reduction in liver enzymes, suggesting a reduction in liver cell injury in the new liver as compared to the group on the regular diet.

The patients on the omega-3 oil also had a significantly shorter hospital stay and significantly fewer complications, especially postoperative infections. Upon a 1-year follow-up of both groups of patients, it was found that three times as many people on the regular diet died as compared to those on the omega-3 diet.

Of the two forms of omega-3 oils, the safest and most effective form appears to be the DHA form, especially the triglyceride formulation of DHA. The Garden of Life DHA supplement has the proper balance and also offers the DHA in the triglyceride form. The dose would be 1000 to 2000 mg a day. Studies have shown DHA improves the tolerance and survival of transplanted organs.

While no direct studies have been done, curcumin has been shown to inhibit the main inflammatory pathways that are activated during transplanted liver rejection, mainly by controlling immune cell receptors (toll-like receptors—such as TLR4). Curcumin also inhibits inflammation in the liver by a number of other mechanisms. The Nano-Curcumin would be the best absorbed and therefore able to get to the liver. Of course, one should consult with their doctor before using either of these compounds.

CHAPTER 18

What to Eat for a Healthy Liver

Your liver depends on you to keep it at peak health. Key to this is eating a healthy diet, since it is your liver that is tasked with metabolizing the foods you eat and drink.

To keep your liver healthy, you must eat a healthy, balanced diet. This is because, when you eat, your digestive system enables food nutrients such as carbohydrates, fats, and proteins to be absorbed into the bloodstream. These nutrients then travel in the blood directly to the liver, where they are processed to either carry out the body's important functions or they are stored.

In addition, it's also your liver's job to neutralize potentially harmful substances—for example, alcohol—and prevent their accumulation in the body.

Thus, maintaining a healthy liver is a prerequisite for preserving overall body homeostasis, which means keeping your body in balance.

Eating for a Healthy or Healing Liver

What to Avoid:

- Foods high in fat, sugar, and salt
- Fried foods
- Omega-6 fats found in margarine, salad dressings, cooking oils, and added to most processed foods; raw or under-cooked shellfish such as oysters and clams; oysters feed by filtering surrounding water where waterborne bacteria (vibrios) may thrive, possibly resulting in the bacteria multiplying in the human body and causing disease.
- Alcohol. If you have liver disease, depending on what type of liver disease you have, you may have to eliminate alcohol altogether. If not, cut it down to one drink a day if you're a woman and two drinks a day if you're a man.

Eat a Balanced Diet

Select foods from all healthy food groups—fruits, vegetables, meats and beans, and healthy oils, such as extra virgin olive oil and coconut oil. Some people do not like the coconut taste. Fortunately, there is a refined form that has no coconut taste or odor.

Eat Food with Fiber

Fiber helps your liver work at an optimal level. Fruits, vegetables, legumes, and oatmeal can take care of your body's fiber needs.

Drink Adequate Amounts of Water, and Drink White or Green Tea

Liquids prevent dehydration, help your liver to function better, and teas supplies your liver with powerful protective compounds.

Diets

There are three different ways of eating that I endorse for their pro-liver benefits. The first is my anti-inflammatory diet, which is excellent for anyone who wants to prevent chronic disease, including those that affect the liver. The DASH diet and the Mediterranean diet also have demonstrated liver benefits.

Dr. Blaylock's Anti-inflammatory Diet

Eat and Drink Vegetables

Eat at least six servings of vegetables a day. These portions should include nutrient-dense ones, such as broccoli, Brussels sprouts, cauliflower, cabbage, onions, leeks, green lettuces, whole tomatoes, collards, mustard greens, spinach, kale, and celery.

Eat the Right Meats

Saturated fats have very little connection to heart disease or cholesterol, despite what your doctor may tell you. However, fats from organically raised meats are much safer than conventionally raised meats, because the latter have fats containing high levels of pesticides, herbicides, industrial chemicals, and toxic metals, and lower beneficial fats. The best diet would include limited amounts of organic chicken, turkey, fish, and some pork (unless restricted by your religion), no more than 6 ounces per day. Grass-fed beef could also be included about once or twice a week. I consider fish in the same category of foods as meat and recommend eating varieties that are low in mercury and high in anti-inflammatory omega-3 fats. Wild salmon is a good choice on both counts. Mercury levels in different fish change over time. The nonprofit Environmental Working Group offers an updated seafood guide at www.ewg.org. While most nutrition sites only talk about seafood mercury levels, also of concern is the pesticide/herbicide levels, which can be quite high in some seafood.

Know Your Fats

Unhealthy, inflammatory fats are omega-6 oils, used as cooking oils, in salad dressings, and in most processed foods. They include corn, safflower, sunflower, peanut, soybean, and canola oils, and should be avoided. These oils oxidize very easily, meaning they degrade, much like how margarine will turn rancid if you leave it outside the refrigerator. They are highly inflammatory within blood vessels, as well as the entire body. They are also known to stimulate cancer growth, invasion, and spread (metastasis). Check labels carefully, because many processed foods use an assortment of these oils.

Some omega-6 fats are essential, but most Western diets contain up to 50 times the amount needed. Vegetables and organically raised meats will supply all the omega-6 fats you need in a much healthier form than the ones in processed foods. Grass-fed cattle have higher healthy omega-3 oils in their meat.

The best cooking oil is extra virgin coconut oil. If you do not like the taste of coconut, use refined coconut oil, which has no odor or taste. For salad dressings, use extra virgin olive oil. Again, be careful of labels. Many commercial brands will have in large letters that the dressing contains "extra virgin olive oil," while in fact it also contains a blend of omega-6 oils.

Drink for Health

Purified water and white or green tea are the best beverages. Water hydrates and cleanses without any liabilities. Hydration is essential for adequate lymphatic flow, one of the more important circulatory systems used to cleanse the body. White and green teas contain antioxidants and anti-inflammatory substances that are therapeutic, as well as hydrating. If you are sensitive to caffeine or find that it keeps you up at night, choose decaffeinated versions. I don't recommend fruit juices because they are high in sugar, fluoride, and, in many cases, aluminum.

Avoid Trans Fats

Listed as "partially hydrogenated" oils, these can be in many processed foods, even if a label claims zero trans fats. That's because food regulations allow a "zero" label if the amount of trans fat is less than 0.5 grams per serving. However, only a few grams of these per day can harm arteries, so eating several servings of foods that contain nearly one-half gram per serving can quickly add up to dangerous amounts. The best way to tell if the food really contains trans fat is to see if any partially hydrogenated oil is listed as an ingredient. Remember, trans fats combined with MSG does great harm to the liver.

Avoid Sugar

The strongest link to heart attacks, strokes, and atherosclerosis is not cholesterol or even fats, but sugar intake. Eliminate, except on special occasions, all sugar products, including cakes, pies, candy, sweetened drinks, fruit juices, and other sugar sources. High-fructose corn syrup should be avoided at all costs, because it is the worst culprit. Read ingredient labels carefully, because this form of sugar is not only in obviously sweet foods but also in many sauces, soups, and other foods we don't normally associate with sugar. Fruits are high in sugar and should be consumed only in limited amounts. Fruit powders with most of the sugar removed is best.

Minimize Starchy Carbohydrates

In the human body, some starches have the same effect as sugar. Foods high in special starches are technically called "high-glycemic" carbohydrates, meaning that they very rapidly convert to blood sugar after being eaten. These include breads (white or whole grain), buns, biscuits, rolls, crackers, chips, cereals, white rice, and potatoes. One should also pay attention to the "glycemic load," that is, the amount of the particular starchy food you are eating. A small amount may be just fine.

Avoid Fluoride

This includes fluorinated water, toothpaste, mouthwash, raisins, other dried fruit, and black tea. Fluoride is a very reactive compound, and even in very small concentrations can damage cells, tissues, and organs. This is especially true in children. The fact that fluoride accumulates in certain tissues of the body makes it especially dangerous.

The DASH Diet

Dietary Approaches to Stop Hypertension, or DASH, is a lifelong approach to healthy eating that's designed to help treat or prevent high blood pressure (hypertension), but has been shown to have numerous other health benefits as well, including for the liver.

What Is the DASH Diet Like?

Here's a look at the recommended servings from each food group for the 2000-calories-a-day DASH diet. While the DASH diet is effective for controlling blood pressure, it contains many items I would not endorse for other reasons.

Grains: 6 to 8 Servings a Day

Grains include bread, cereal, rice, and pasta. Examples of one serving of grains include 1 slice of whole-wheat bread, 1 ounce of dry cereal, or ½ cup of cooked cereal, rice, or pasta. I do not endorse the eating of grains, at least not regularly. They are high in lectins, which damage tissues, and many are high in the excitotoxin glutamate. Most are also high in gluten.

Vegetables: 4 to 5 Servings a Day

Tomatoes, carrots, broccoli, sweet potatoes, greens, and other vegetables are full of fiber, vitamins, and such minerals as potassium and magnesium. Examples of one serving includes 1 cup of raw leafy green vegetables or ½ cup of cut-up raw or cooked vegetables. Tomatoes are high in glutamate and lectins. Glutamate is especially of concern in tomato sauces and purees.

Fruits: 4 to 5 Servings a Day

Like vegetables, fruits are packed with fiber, potassium, extremely benefical flavonoids, and magnesium and are typically low in fat (coconuts are an exception). They are high in sugar (fructose).

Examples of one serving include one medium fruit, ½ cup of fresh, frozen, or canned fruit, or 4 ounces of juice.

Some citrus fruits and juices, such as grapefruit, can interact with certain medications, so check with your doctor or pharmacist to see if they're OK for you.

Whole organic fruits are generally preferred to juices, and if they have edible peels, leave them on because the peel is fiber-filled. All fruits should be washed with a veggie wash before eating, even organically grown. The healthiest fruits include strawberries, blueberries, and raspberries.

Dairy: 2 to 3 Servings a Day

Milk, yogurt, cheese, and other dairy products are major sources of calcium, vitamin D, and protein. Low-fat is preferable. This has been removed from the more modern DASH diet. Milk should never be consumed in any form, as it can stimulate cancer growth, especially prostate cancer. This is because of the high calcium content. Cow's milk also has relatively high glutamate levels and is a high allergic food. Never drink soy milk as it has damaging effects on the brain and is high in fluoride, aluminum, and glutamate.

Lean Meat, Poultry, and Fish: Six 1-Ounce Servings, or Fewer, a Day

Meat can be a rich source of protein, B vitamins, iron, and zinc. Choose a variety of meat and aim for no more than four to six 1-ounce servings a day.

One can trim away the fat should they so choose, but it is not essential. Bake, broil, grill, or roast instead of frying it a cooking oil. Avoid all soybean products.

Heart-Healthy Fish, such as Salmon, Herring, and Tuna

These types of fish are high in omega-3 fatty acids, which are healthy for your heart. Only buy "Safe Catch" tuna or other brands that have been tested and cleared of mercury contamination. Make sure the fish is not from fish farms. Many brands will say "Wild" on the label, but they are farmed raised.

Nuts, Seeds, and Legumes: 4 to 5 Servings a Week

Almonds, sunflower seeds, kidney beans, peas, lentils, and other foods in this family are good sources of magnesium, potassium, and protein. Be careful of the amount you consume and how often, as nuts are higher in calories, omega-6 oils, and glutamate.

Examples of one serving include ⅓ cup of nuts, 2 tablespoons of seeds or nut butter, or ½ cup of cooked beans or peas.

Fats and Oils: 2 to 3 Servings a Day

The DASH diet strives for a healthy balance by limiting total fat to less than 30% of daily calories, with a focus on the healthier monounsaturated fats. This has been disproven. It is the omega-6 fats that are most harmful. One can consume higher than 30% fats as long as they reduce their carbohydrate intake.

The Mediterranean Diet

Countless studies attest to the health benefits of the Mediterranean diet, which is based on the way people ate in such countries as Greece and Italy in the 1960s. The people living there have the lowest rates of chronic problems, including heart disease and cancer, and now some studies show that this way of eating is also excellent for liver health.

Foods that rarely—if ever—appear on the Mediterranean diet include deli meats, hot dogs, sausages, cookies, cakes, pies, brownies, ice cream, and other desserts, or sugary drinks. People who follow the Mediterranean diet also rarely eat processed trans fats such as margarine, refined oils (soy, cottonseed, and canola), and processed foods that contain those oils. Their primary source of fat comes from olive oil.

The following are the foods from which people on the Mediterranean diet build their menus:

- **Vegetables.** Broccoli, kale, spinach, onions, cauliflower, carrots, Brussels sprouts, cucumbers, etc.
- **Fruits.** Strawberries, blueberries, raspberries, blackberries, apples, bananas, oranges, pears, grapes, dates, figs, melons, peaches, etc. These are all high in fructose and should be eaten in limited amounts. Fruit powders devoid of sugar are best.
- **Nuts and seeds.** Almonds, walnuts, macadamia nuts, hazelnuts, cashews, sunflower seeds, pumpkin seeds, etc. Again, some are high in omega-6 oils and glutamate.

- **Legumes.** Beans, peas, lentils, pulses, peanuts, chickpeas, etc. Must be well cooked as all are high in lectins.
- **Tubers.** Potatoes, sweet potatoes, turnips, yams, etc. Irish potatoes are on the high glycemic list.
- **Whole grains.** Whole oats, brown rice, rye, barley, corn, buckwheat, whole wheat, whole-grain bread, and pasta. Again, these are high in gluten, glutamate, and lectins.
- **Fish and seafood.** Salmon, sardines, trout, tuna, mackerel, shrimp, oysters, clams, crab, mussels. Eat only low or mercury-free seafood.
- **Poultry.** Chicken, duck, turkey, etc. Only organically raised.
- **Eggs.** Chicken, quail, duck eggs. (Organic)
- **Dairy.** Cheese, yogurt, Greek yogurt, etc. Avoid all of these.
- **Herbs and spices.** Garlic, basil, mint, rosemary, sage, nutmeg, cinnamon, pepper, etc.
- **Healthy fats.** Extra virgin olive oil, olives, avocados, and olive oil.
- **Beverages.** Water is recommended as the main beverage. A moderate amount of red wine (about one glass a day) is allowed. This is optional and should be avoided by anyone who has problems with alcohol or liver disease or damage. Coffee and white or green tea are acceptable, but avoid sugar-sweetened beverages or fruit juices. Use no artificial sweeteners except monk fruit juice.

Eating Gluten-free May Benefit Your Liver

Gluten, which is a mixture of two proteins, and most commonly found in wheat, can be difficult to digest for some people, especially those with celiac disease and gluten sensitivity, as discussed in Chapter 3.

If you have celiac disease, eating gluten-free is a must. But it is also preferable if you've found that you are sensitive to foods made with gluten. Gluten in excess is harmful to everyone, not just the "gluten sensitive" person. Modern processed foods add additional gluten above that found naturally.

The most cost-effective and healthy way to follow the gluten-free diet is to seek out these naturally gluten-free food groups, which include:

- Fruits
- Vegetables
- Meat and poultry
- Fish
- Beans, legumes, and nuts

Pure wheatgrass and barley grass are gluten-free, but there is gluten in the seeds. If they are not harvested or processed correctly, there is risk of gluten contamination.

On a gluten-free diet, you avoid grain products that contain gluten, but that doesn't mean you can't enjoy rice, millet, quinoa, and buckwheat, which are just a few examples. In addition, there are gluten-free pastas today made from corn, quinoa, beans, and other vegetables, including cauliflower and zucchini. All vegetables should be certified as GMO free.

You also have to play detective, because gluten, much like sugar, lurks in foods you wouldn't expect, including energy bars, French fries, soup, soy sauce, salad dressings, and many more. While food companies are required to list allergens on the label (e.g., eggs, nuts), they are not required to do this with gluten. So, even if a food says "gluten-free" on the label, you need to read the ingredients.

Check out the Celiac Disease Foundation for a wealth of information on their website, including food lists covering items such as beverages, candy bars, and other products, as well as meal plans, information on ingredients, and much, much more (www.celiac.org).

Special Recommendations for Those with Liver Disease

If you have liver disease, your condition may require special nutritional considerations. Here are some general considerations regarding major types of liver disease. For less common liver diseases, or instructions on any type of liver disease you have, it's important to check with your doctor.

Alcohol-Related Liver Disease

If you have been drinking alcohol excessively, an early stage of liver disease is the buildup of fatty deposits. This can be reversed completely, if you abstain from alcohol. Approximately 20% of people with alcohol-related fatty liver disease go on to develop alcoholic hepatitis and eventually cirrhosis.

Also, if you have alcohol-related liver disease or damage, you may be malnourished, meaning you aren't consuming all of the nutrients your body requires. You may still be malnourished even if you are overweight, depending on what you eat, how you eat, or if your weight is increased because your body is retaining fluid.

The most important change to your diet you can make is to stop drinking alcohol. Eating a balanced diet, with sufficient protein, healthy fats, and carbohydrates, is essential.

People who are malnourished due to alcohol-related liver disease may particularly lack the vitamin thiamine (a B vitamin that helps the body convert carbohydrates into energy). Benfotiamine is the best compound to raise vitamin B1 levels, as the B1 levels persist longer than taking vitamin B1 itself. This compound also has additional benefits as well. Taking it along with the vitamin form may be even better. You should be prescribed B vitamins if you are drinking alcohol at harmful levels, or are alcohol-dependent, or if you are malnourished or at risk of becoming so. A multi–B vitamin is best.

Hepatitis

If you have acute hepatitis, you may feel quite well, and should try to eat a healthy liver diet, as described in the general recommendations earlier, unless your condition causes you to become nauseous and makes eating difficult.

Chronic Viral Hepatitis

If you have a long-term hepatitis infection (where the infection lasts longer than 6 months) caused by a virus such as hepatitis B, you should eat a normal diet that is healthy for your liver. If you are losing weight, though, consult your doctor. You should also avoid all types of diets that require you to fast or skip meals.

Fatty Liver Disease

If you have nonalcoholic fatty liver disease, a key to managing your condition is weight loss. Even dropping just 5% of your body weight could lower the fat in your liver. Lose between 7 and 10% of your body weight and you'll lower inflammation and the odds of injury to your liver cells. You might even reverse some of the damage. Go slow: 1 to 2 pounds per week is fine.

There are guidelines on which foods to avoid if you have fatty liver disease, and just following them could very well result in weight loss.

In addition, research has found that the DASH diet and the Mediterranean diet, explained earlier, have been shown to help reverse nonalcoholic fatty liver disease. I recommend my modified form of these diets for even better results.

In research published in *International Liver*, 60 overweight and obese patients with nonalcoholic fatty liver disease were randomly allocated to either the control diet or the DASH diet for 8 weeks. Both diets restricted calories and both diets consisted of 52 to 55% carbohydrates, 16 to 18% proteins, and 30% total fats. However, the DASH diet was high in fruits, vegetables, whole grains, low-fat dairy products, and were low in saturated fats, cholesterol, and refined grains.

After 8 weeks, the DASH diet group showed significant improvements in liver function test results, weight, body mass index, insulin resistance issues, insulin sensitivity, triglyceride levels, total/HDL cholesterol ratio, and hs-CRP, a measure of inflammation. Some of the markers that show liver stress were also improved in the DASH diet group.

The Mediterranean diet is also an excellent way to reduce your risk of fatty liver disease because it targets a number of conditions that comprise the metabolic syndrome, a collection of conditions that steeply hike fatty liver risk.

One recent study, for example, looked at 1521 middle-aged and older people who closely followed a Mediterranean-style diet for 6 years. They were at significantly lower risk of developing fatty liver disease than others in a large prospective study.

Individuals whose diets improved the most had about 80% less liver fat accumulation between baseline and follow-up compared with those whose diets worsened the most.

More Tips on Eating for Liver Health

How to Kick the Sugar Habit

First off, cut out the obvious offenders. Banish the sugar bowl, soft drinks, candy, etc., from your house, car, and office! Then follow these tips:

- Make sure you're actually hungry, not thirsty. Sugar cravings can be a sign you're dehydrated.
- Get enough sleep. Research finds that people who are tired tend to crave junk foods, including sugar.
- Eat more protein. Consuming protein in all three meals can help beat down sugar cravings. Eggs, chicken, fish, and even modest amounts of red meat are all good ways to pump up the protein.
- Banish alcohol. Not only is it bad for your liver, but cocktails are packed with sugar, and booze can weaken your resolve to lay off other sweet items.
- If your sweet tooth absolutely craves a fix, eat a few small squares of dark chocolate. The higher the percentage of dark chocolate in the product, the lower the sugar content, as opposed to milk chocolate, which contains added sugar and fat.

Liver Power Foods

The following foods are especially nourishing to the liver:

Apples

Fruits are good for the liver in general, and apples are especially a powerhouse. They contain chemicals called *polyphenols* that help keep fats in the blood under control, as well as pectin and malic acid that help remove toxins and carcinogens. In addition, they have anti-inflammatory properties that protect you against fatty liver disease. Purchase only organically grown apples and wash them with a veggie wash.

Artichokes

Artichokes are rich in luteolin, cynarine, chlorogenic acid, and other compounds that enhance the liver's detoxification mechanism, protect against oxidation, and reduce liver damage risk. They are also high in inulin, which stimulates components of the immune system and is a food for the probiotics in your colon.

Avocados

Fatty foods are bad for the liver, but one fat that is beneficial is the type contained in avocados. Research finds that moderate consumption of avocados, as part of a balanced diet, was associated with weight loss and overall improved liver function tests. They also showed people had a lower body mass index, smaller waist circumference, and higher levels of HDL (good) cholesterol.

Beets and Beetroot Juice

Beetroot juice protects the liver from inflammation and enhances its natural detoxification enzymes. Beets and beet juice are high in nitrates, which can raise nitric oxide levels which is harmful in cases of several liver disorders, especially cirrhosis.

Blueberries

High in antioxidants and fiber, blueberries are one of nature's healthiest fruits. In terms of the liver, some research suggests that blueberries may help protect against liver damage and reduce the risk of fibrosis, or excessive connective tissue within the liver. mainly by their very high content of pterostilbene. Research also finds cranberries to be liver healthy as well. Blueberry powder devoid of sugar is best.

Broccoli

Along with other cruciferous vegetables, such as cauliflower, Brussels sprouts, cabbage, and kale, broccoli is rich in sulforaphane and other compounds that boost detoxification and protect the liver from damage.

Coffee

Several studies have found that coffee can benefit the liver by protecting it against fatty liver disease and lowering the risk of cirrhosis, and may also protect it against liver cancer. Also, a study in the *Journal of Gastroenterology* in 2014 suggested that the beneficial effects of coffee might be due to how it influences liver enzymes. However, because coffee contains caffeine, which is a stimulant, you should drink it sparingly or choose decaffeinated brands.

Fatty Fish

Fish is a great source of protein, and fatty fish is rich in omega-3 fatty acids, the good type of fats that help reduce inflammation. These fats may be especially helpful in the liver, as they appear to prevent the buildup of excess fats and maintain enzyme levels in the liver. In addition, there is research that suggests that eating fish may help lower the risk of liver cancer. Avoid fish high in mercury, such as tuna (Safe Catch is clean), shark, swordfish, tile fish, and redfish. Sardines are completely safe and an excellent source of omega-3 oils. They should be packed in olive oil, not water.

Garlic

Adding garlic to the diet may also help stimulate the liver. A 2016 study in the journal *Advanced Biomedical Research* notes that garlic consumption reduces body weight and fat content in people with NAFLD, with no changes to lean body mass. This is beneficial, as being overweight or obese is a contributing factor to NAFLD.

Grapefruit

Grapefruit is high in naringin, which is metabolized as naringenin, an antioxidant that also helps protect the liver against inflammation. Some animal studies suggest naringin may reduce the risk of cirrhosis and hepatic fibrosis, the development of excessive connective tissue in the liver. Check with your doctor to make sure that grapefruit doesn't interact with any prescription drugs you may be taking, as it inhibits certain phase I detoxification enzymes. It can prolong the stimulating effect of coffee.

Grapes

Grapes, particularly red and purple ones (the colors are made by pigments that are high in antioxidants), are generally considered healthful to the liver, but some are high in fluoride. Animal studies find a number of benefits, including reducing inflammation and preventing cellular damage. In addition, a small study on humans found grape seed extract improved liver function in non-alcoholic fatty liver disease. There is a Nano-Grape Seed extract that is highly absorbable.

Nuts

Generally healthful, nuts typically contain unsaturated fatty acids, vitamin E, polyphenois, and antioxidants. These compounds may help prevent fatty liver disease, as well as reduce inflammation and oxidative stress. They are high in glutamate, and some have omega-6 oils. They should be eaten in limited amounts.

Oatmeal

Oatmeal is also rich in fiber, which helps the liver function optimally. Furthermore, oats and oatmeal are high in compounds called *beta-glucans*, which are particularly helpful to the liver. They help balance the immune system, reduce inflammation, and may help prevent diabetes. In addition, some preliminary animal research suggests they may help reduce the amount of fat stored in the liver. But don't opt for prepackaged oatmeal, which may contain fillers or sugar; choose whole or steel-cut oats.

Olive Oil

Eating too much fat is not good for the liver, but some fats may help it. According to a *World Journal of Gastroenterology* study, adding olive oil to the diet may help reduce oxidative stress and improve liver function. This is due to the high content of mono unsaturated fatty acids in the oil. Countries having very low cancer rates and high general health and longevity consume a great deal of olive oil.

Teas

Drinking tea is generally healthy, and there are benefits specific to the liver as well. Black, green, and white teas are overall found to be healthy, but I am a particular proponent of white and green teas, which can improve your health in many ways. The difference between white and green tea is that white tea is picked as a younger plant than green tea, and it has a higher content of these beneficial chemicals and lower levels of aluminum and fluoride. For its part, green tea may contain special benefits for the liver, including reducing fat, fighting against oxidative stress, and benefiting people with fatty liver disease. Black tea has a high content of fluoride and aluminum.

Supplements for General Liver Health

These supplements aid liver health in general. Others for specific diseases are mentioned in the appropriate chapters.

Quercetin

Quercetin protects the lining of the stomach and intestines from damage, mainly by inhibiting inflammation and neutralizing free radicals. It also reduces inflammation. Quercetin is oil soluble. Nano-Quercetin is far better absorbed that raw quercetin.

What to do. Take 250 mg of Nano-Quercetin three times daily.

Taurine

This sulfur-containing amino acid, which has been shown to improve detoxification systems, can cause a drop in blood sugar in people with reactive hypoglycemia. Such individuals should take tablets or capsules with meals.

What to do. Take 500 mg 30 minutes before a meal, two or three times a day.

R-Lipoic Acid

This compound, also called *thioctic acid*, is found naturally in all cells and tissues of the body, and is a very powerful and versatile antioxidant. It also greatly improves the ability of the liver and cells to detoxify important environmental poisons.

What to do. Take 100 mg twice a day with a meal for general protection, and as high as 600 mg three times a day for those at high risk because of diabetes.

Silymarin

A compound isolated from the milk thistle plant, silymarin has shown a tremendous ability to improve detoxification, even when a person has been exposed to powerful liver toxins.

What to do. The dose is 200 mg a day for general maintenance, and 200 to 400 mg, three times a day, when heavily exposed to toxins.

Resources

A Word About Health Foundations

Unfortunately, health foundations, in general, have several drawbacks. First is that most are in the business of health and not actual innovative health science. Many studies analyzing such foundations find that much of the money goes for things other than actual scientific research in their cited disease. Second, and most important, they are severely constrained in terms of innovative information, especially natural treatments, as they need to avoid criticism from orthodox medical institutions. Such criticism could ruin their reputation in the media. The research I present in this book is backed by scientific studies, admittedly much of which is based on using animal models of human disease, with a number involving clinical studies. A significant number of people have tried these innovative treatments on their own and report excellent results. The compounds I discuss have all had extensive safety testing. Natural products have far less side effects than pharmaceutical drugs, especially in terms of deaths and severe side effects. In my opinion, government-based medical associations are the least reliable. I list some of them for completeness' sake.

General Organizations

Celiac Disease Foundation
20350 Ventura Blvd. Ste. 240
Woodland Hills, CA 91364
Tel: 818-716-1513
Fax: 818-267-5577
Helpline: 818-716-1513, Ext. 110
www.celiac.org

Specialized Resources

Alcoholism and Substance Abuse
National Institute on Alcohol Abuse and Alcoholism (NIAAA)
Tel: 301-443-3860
www.niaaa.nih.gov

Genetic Diseases

Hemochromatosis
Iron Disorders Institute
P.O. Box 4891
Greenville, SC 29608
info@irondisorders.org
Hemochromatosis.org

Wilson Disease Organization
5572 N Diversey Blvd
Milwaukee, WI 53217
Tel: 414-961-0533
Fax: 414-962-3886, TDD: 540-743-1415
info@wilsondisease.org

Hepatitis

Autoimmune Hepatitis Foundation
https://www.aihep.org/
Email: info@aihep.org

Hepatitis Foundation International
504 Blick Drive
Silver Spring, MD
Tel: 800-891-0707
Email: info@hepatitisfoundation.org

Liver Cancer

Books

- *Natural Strategies for Cancer Patients*
  Russell L. Blaylock, M.D. Citadel (revised and updated), 2019
- *Grain Brain*
  David Perlmutter, M.D. Little, Brown Spark, 2018
- *Health and Nutrition Secrets*
  Russell L. Blaylock, M.D., Health Press, 2006
- *Dr. Blaylock's Prescriptions for Natural Health*
  Humanix Books, 2016

Newsletters

I write a monthly newsletter, *The Blaylock Wellness Report*, on the subject of natural health in which I discuss various health issues in detail. Subscribers get access to all back issues. All main subjects are fully referenced with scientific citations.

- *Artificial Sweeteners: The Bad, the Worse, and the Downright Deadly*, June 2021
- *Our Bodies' Invisible Creatures*, August 2012 (about probiotics)
- *Managing Iron and Other Potential Deadly Toxins*, August 2019
- *Taurine: The Miracle Amino Acid*, December 2016
- *Prevent the Top Destroyer of Good Health: Inflammation*, September 2014
- *Magnesium Deficiency Is Widespread, Untreated . . . And Deadly*, July 2011
- *Diabetes Cure: What you Need to Know*, January 2015
- *Natural Treatments That Prevent and Cure Deadly Colon Cancer*, September 2015
- *Revealed: The Food Industry's Deadly Lies About Fat*, May 2013

Blue Faery: The Adrienne Wilson Liver Cancer Association
1919 Oxmoor Rd #257
Birmingham, AL 35209
Phone: 818-636-5624
Email: andrea@bluefaery.org

Smart Patients: Liver Cancer Community
info@smartpatients.com
www.smartpatients.com

Liver Transplantation

National Foundation for Transplants
3249 W. Sarazen's Cir., Ste. 100
Memphis, TN 38125
Toll free: (800) 489-3863. Local: (901) 684-1697
info@transplants.org

Scientific Registrar of Transplant Recipients
www.srtr.org

United Network for Organ Sharing (UNOS)
Patient info: (888) 894-6361
www.unos.org

Acknowledgments

I would like to thank Chris Ruddy, the owner of Newsmax publications and Newsmax TV, for all his help in making this book possible. I thank the staff of Humanix Books for all their valuable help in making this book a reality and of the highest quality. A special thanks to Mary Glenn, publisher of Humanix Books, for her kindness and valuable assistance, and Charlotte Libov for her diligence and hard work in putting this book together.

Above all I thank the Lord for His guidance in all that I do. It is His guidance that sustains us all and leads us on the right path in life.

Index

About the Author

Dr. Blaylock is a retired, board-certified neurosurgeon, who received his medical education at Louisiana State University School of Medicine, graduating in 1971. He completed a surgical internship at the Medical University of South Carolina from 1971 to 1972. During that time, he trained under Dr. Curtis Arts and Dr. John Moncrief, two of the world's top experts in burns and trauma.

From 1972 to 1977, Dr. Blaylock completed his neurosurgical residency at the Medical University of South Carolina directed by Dr. Phanor Perot. He also trained with Dr. Ludwig Kempe, a world-renowned neurosurgeon and author of the then classic, two-volume *Illustrated Neurosurgical Text*. Along with Dr. Kempe, Dr. Blaylock developed the transcollosal removal of intraventricular meningiomas, and presented a paper on the technique at the Congress of Neurological Surgeons international meeting in 1976.

Dr. Blaylock was board certified in neurological surgery in 1977. He became a member of the American Association of Neurological Surgeons in 1980, and was board certified in clinical nutrition in 2007.

Dr. Blaylock was appointed to the editorial board of the journal *Fluoride* and to the *Journal of American Physicians and Surgeons* and has now retired from both. Presently he holds the position of associate editor-in-chief of the neuroinflammatory section of the journal *Surgical Neurology International* and is on the editorial staff of the neuropsychiatry section of the same journal. For two years, Dr. Blaylock was a lectuter for the certification program of the Foundation for Anti-Aging Medicine and Regenerative Medicine.

He has published 60 scientific and opinion articles for peer-reviewed journals on a variety of subjects, including cancer, the cytokine storm, Parkinson's disease, chronic traumatic encephalopathy, nutritional medicine, autism spectrum disorders, Gulf-war syndrome, and neurodevelopmental toxicology of aluminum, fluoride, and mercury. Dr. Blaylock has written or cowritten six books, wrote chapters for four books, and wrote introductions for a number of books on health subjects.

In addition, Dr. Blaylock is an accomplished professional artist and writes a monthly newsletter, the *Blaylock Wellness Newsletter*. He is married and has two children and four grandchildren (one in Heaven).

Simple **Heart Test**

Powered by Newsmaxhealth.com

FACT:

▸ Nearly half of those who die from heart attacks each year never showed prior symptoms of heart disease.

▸ If you suffer cardiac arrest outside of a hospital, you have just a 7% chance of survival.

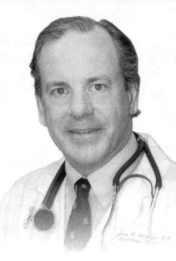

Don't be caught off guard. Know your risk now.

TAKE THE TEST NOW ...

Renowned cardiologist **Dr. Chauncey Crandall** has partnered with **Newsmaxhealth.com** to create a simple, easy-to-complete, online test that will help you understand your heart attack risk factors. Dr. Crandall is the author of the #1 best-seller *The Simple Heart Cure: The 90-Day Program to Stop and Reverse Heart Disease.*

Take Dr. Crandall's Simple Heart Test — it takes just 2 minutes or less to complete — it could save your life!

Discover your risk now.

- **Where you score on our unique heart disease risk scale**
- Which of your lifestyle habits really protect your heart
- **The true role your height and weight play in heart attack risk**
- Little-known conditions that impact heart health
- **Plus much more!**

SimpleHeartTest.com/24

Improve Memory and Sharpen Your Mind

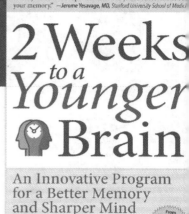

"Gary Small is the expert to listen to if you're concerned about your memory." —*Jerome Yesavage, MD, Stanford University School of Medical*

2 Weeks *to a* Younger Brain

An Innovative Program for a Better Memory and Sharper Mind

GARY SMALL, MD
DIRECTOR, UCLA LONGEVITY CENTER
and GIGI VORGAN

From the authors of *New York Times* best-seller *The Memory Bible*

> **FREE OFFER**

Misplacing your keys, forgetting someone's name at a party, or coming home from the market without the most important item — these are just some of the many common memory slips we all experience from time to time.

Most of us laugh about these occasional memory slips, but for some, it's no joke. Are these signs of dementia, or worse, Alzheimer's? Dr. Garry Small will help dissuade those fears and teach you practical strategies and exercises to sharpen your mind in his breakthrough book, *2 Weeks To A Younger Brain*.

This book will show that it only takes two weeks to form new habits that bolster cognitive abilities and help stave off or even reverse brain aging.

If you commit only 14 days to *2 Weeks To A Younger Brain*, you will reap noticeable results. During that brief period, you will have learned the secrets of keeping your brain young for the rest of your life.

Claim Your FREE OFFER Now!

Claim your **FREE** copy of *2 Weeks To A Younger Brain* — a $19.99 value — today with this special offer. Just cover $4.95 for shipping & handling.

Plus, you will receive a 3-month risk-free trial subscription to *The Mind Health Report*. Every issue of *The Mind Health Report* is filled with the latest advancements and breakthrough techniques for improving & enhancing your memory, brain health and longevity. **That's a $29 value, yours FREE!**

Claim Your FREE Book With This Special Offer!
Newsmax.com/24